Spindoctor

ROY RICKMAN

FORD CROSS BOOKS

First published in 2006 by

Ford Cross Books
P.O. Box 135
Bideford, Devon
EX39 9AN

ISBN 0 955 3360 0 7
ISBN 978_0_9553360 0 3

Typesetting by: Thurbans Publishing Services, Farnham, Surrey

Cover design: David Porteous Editions, Newton Abbot

Production by: Richard Joseph Publishers Ltd, PO Box 15,
Torrington EX38 8ZJ

Printed by: Ashford Colour Press Ltd, Gosport, Hampshire PO13 0FW

Dedication

This book is dedicated to my wife Shirley Patricia and to our three children, Karen, Alistair and Graeme – whose patient tolerance and understanding, of my many absences from them, made it possible.

David Shepherd.

with the best wishes and
compliments of the author

Roy Rickerman
November 2006.

As promised earlier –
pages 54 and 230 refer –
no acknowledgement needed.

best wishes

Roy Rickerman.

'I speak of Africa and golden joys'

– Henry IV, Part II, Act.V, Scene 3

Contents

Illustrations

CHAPTER 1

Waiting for 'Mr. Whiskers'

The leopard came just before midnight. We didn't see or hear it of course, although we had been waiting for its arrival since dusk, sitting precariously and in considerable discomfort on the top of a small open coupé, with its front jacked up some 3-4 feet in the air. Our rifles were supposedly at the ready – but ready for what wasn't exactly clear to either of us. Our ludicrously inept and inadequate preparations for its demise, and with the car in this 'sit-up-and-beg' position, were enough to make any self-respecting big-cat fall about laughing; it's a wonder we didn't hear it – we could have made a fortune as a music-hall turn.

Ostensibly we were waiting for it to return to its kill, the headless body of what, until that afternoon, had been a large and affectionate Airedale dog, but which was now wedged firmly in the fork of a large straight tree some 25 yards in front of us. To illuminate our intended target we had trained the car headlights on to the body of the dog. To do this we had adopted the dubious expedient of lifting the front of the car, to what seemed an impossible height, with a huge 'Tanganyika' jack, an impressive heavy-duty device designed to lift grossly overladen lorries, mostly in the rainy season, out of East Africa's notoriously glutinous black-cotton soil.

With the car at this acute angle absolute immobility was essential if we weren't to rock it off the jack and come down to earth with a crash. But this delicate balance was constantly endangered by our frequent and largely ineffectual swipes at the mosquitoes whining round our ears. Understandably, somewhat oblivious of the magical night noises of the African bush, I began seriously to consider whether I wouldn't have a more promising career elsewhere.

My thoughts involuntarily turned to wondering what physical effects would result from a doubtless determined assault by a very athletic and angry big cat, supposing we were, by chance, to hit it; but not for long. Mentally visualising the impressive musculature and 'piano-in-the-mouth' dentition of the average adult African leopard, I quickly abandoned what was clearly not a very reassuring line of thought! My companion, an ex-trainee Gurkha officer, seemed completely unconcerned. The .22 calibre rifle resting across my knees looked (and sadly was) unreassuringly inadequate and I felt myself hoping that my companion's fine 8mm rifle was accurately 'sighted in'; his previous experience with the Gurkhas was the best possible guarantee that he knew how to use it!

Donald, my companion, was a heavily bearded, well-qualified and experienced medical entomologist at the London School of Hygiene & Tropical Medicine. Having obtained a grant from the British Medical Research Council in London, he had recently arrived in Kenya to study the sand-fly (*Phlebotomus*) vectors of 'Kala-azar' (visceral leishmaniasis). This is a major tropical disease, lethal when untreated, the parasites (known as Leishman-Donovan or 'LD' bodies) invading and killing the white blood cells producing severe anaemia and destroying the body's natural defences against bacteria and other infections. With no such illustrious pedigree, I had recently accepted a 5-year contract with the Kenya Medical Department, to make a modest start with the Division of Insect-borne Diseases in Nairobi, as a very junior Entomological Field Officer, where it quickly became apparent that I had much to be modest about and almost everything still to learn. I had obtained this opportunity on the strength of 3 'A' levels in natural sciences hardly won at night school whilst working as a cartographical surveyor with H.M. Ordnance Survey in outer London.

When first accepted for this post I concluded that the representatives of H.M. Crown Agents for the Colonies who interviewed me, must either have been desperate for field staff or, even more unlikely, had seen in me a promising reservoir of research potential that had escaped the notice of everyone else – myself included. Still, the work promised to be interesting; it might one day lead to a scientifically lucrative career in tropical medicine and conjured up heady visions of dedicated scientists looking earnestly down microscopes (doubtless to the background music of jungle drums) to find miracle cures for dread diseases – a useful subject for exploration by Tarzan-oriented film-script writers. However, return to mundane reality clearly indicated that, with no proper qualifications and with only a 3-month crash-course in tropical laboratory technology at the 'London School of Hygiene & Tropical Medicine', there was no alternative but to start at the bottom – in the deep end. Just how deep this was I would soon find out – providing our guardian angels were awake and of a mind to lend a helping hand in our present impending predicament.

Soon after out arrival in Kenya, Donald had rented the vacant half of a pleasant cottage situated in a secluded spot in the middle of a beautiful wood, some way back from the main road at Langata, on the outskirts of Nairobi and adjoining the Game Park. Occupying the other half of the house was the owner M.Chmeilinski, a retired Polish consular official, who spent much of his time playing the ‘cello, often accompanied at the piano by his equally talented wife. Being so close to the perimeter fence of the Nairobi National Park, wild animals wandered through the gardens at will and at night these became a virtual safari park. Hyaenas raiding the dustbins was an almost nightly occurrence – the flash of green eyes and the sloping back in the torch beam made identification easy. This was invariably confirmed by their derisive ‘whooo-oop’ to the badly directed brickbat and the shuffling lope as they departed the scene. In the Karen and Langata districts of Nairobi, with the forest and the proximity of the ‘Athi Plains’ nearby, leopards were a perennial problem. Dogs were always a favoured item on their menu and had little chance against the power, speed and sheer ferocity of these most dangerous of big cats.

Elinor van Someren, the mosquito entomologist at the Division of Insect-borne Diseases (DIBD), who had lived at Karen for many years with her husband Chum and family, had lost a whole succession of dogs, of all sizes and shapes, to leopards over the years. Although lions frequently came into their garden at night, mainly to drink from their small lake, they had never troubled any of their domestic pets – although one must suppose these would have maintained a very low profile on such occasions! One afternoon Donald and I arrived back from the Medical Research Laboratories at about 5 p.m., to find Mr. Chmeilinski anxious about the apparent disappearance of his dog. Earlier that afternoon he had heard a short yelp but, on going out on to the verandah to see, could find no trace of the dog. A few spots of dried blood on the floor, however, provided the first tacit evidence of what must have occurred. We promised to help find the dog: that was our first mistake!

Donald started searching the sides and back of the house. I opted to look along the paths in the front and very soon came to a spot where the foliage at the edge of the path was very dense. Parting the vegetation with my hands I thrust my head through for a better look. In front of my eyes, some 10 ft away, was the smooth trunk of what seemed to be a large unbranched tree. At its foot, half-hidden in the long grass and seemingly still wearing a look of pained surprise and indignation, was the partly chewed head of the neighbour’s luckless Airedale dog.

As I started to lift my head to see further up the tree, one small item of long-stored and generally useless information floated up to consciousness – "leopards only attack man when mutual eye contact has been made". My back hair rose and I froze momentarily. But curiosity won. Looking up, my gaze swept up the limbless trunk to the body of the dog, some 20 ft above the ground, neatly placed in the main fork of the tree. There was no leopard; I resumed normal breathing. Claw marks at regular intervals showed the path of the leopard, where, with the 30 kg body in its mouth, it had swept straight up the trunk in one bound and with what must have been an awesome display of physical power. I backed out of the shrubbery to call my companions.

Soon after our arrival in Kenya, and taking advantage of the Government's assisted purchase facility, I had bought a second-hand Fiat 500 ('Topolino') car. By chance Donald had purchased a similar model. Since they were not very heavy, had good headlights and a fold-down canvas roof they were ideally suited for the task of providing some light relief for, in a temporary fit of insanity, we had decided to sit out over the kill and put an end to 'Mr. Whiskers'. That was our second mistake. Having cut away enough of the surrounding vegetation the next obvious task was to fetch suitable tools for the job in hand. I bravely resisted the temptation to ask 'mine host' if he happened to have an old, but serviceable, anti-tank gun available (which I could have fired over open sights with some hope of success). To my inexpert eye both our weapons looked somewhat inadequate and did little to allay my now mounting misgivings!

So far as I knew, Donald had won no prizes at Bisley; my only previous claim to fame, as a marksman of distinction, was the sole occasion during early RAF aircrew training when, on a practice range, I had accidentally put all 10 bullets through the bullseye and won a £5 sweepstake – much to my surprise and that of my companions. But this was of surprisingly little comfort to me now! At sundown, now fully equipped with sandwiches and flasks of hot coffee, we had climbed up into the car with a degree of caution similar to that adopted by Mt. Everest mountaineers negotiating the final rock band. We settled down to await the arrival of 'Mr. Whiskers'. The first interruption came only minutes later. A babble of excited voices coming up the footpath, behind us in the bush, accompanied by bangings and crashings announced the arrival of a 'support group' – dragging a huge lion trap.

The group was headed by the world-famous anthropologist Dr. Louis Leakey and members of his family and staff who lived nearby. Armand and Michaela Denis, of early TV wildlife fame, were other celebrity neighbours. This trap was on loan from the Kenya Game Department (Nairobi National Park) and was an impressive affair with strong metal bars, a solid wooden floor and a heavily reinforced drop door. A long iron rod linked the door with a baited arm in the centre of the cage. Pulling the bait disengaged the rod allowing the door to drop. Dr. Leakey provided some encouragement by saying “This trap has never caught anything but you might as well try it. But do be careful – leopards can be very dangerous animals you know”. The trap was duly set up some 10 or so yards behind us in thick bush and baited with a huge haunch of meat. This completed, the party took its leave of us, the footsteps and voices faded away and we were once again left to enjoy the persistent attentions of the local mosquito hordes to the accompaniment of a ‘continuo of crickets’ and the ‘pink-pink’ of the tiny tree frogs. As we sat there quietly listening for any sound of Mr. Whiskers’ approach, time went into slow-motion mode and I found myself thinking back over the circumstances that had collectively conspired to bring me to this most unlikely of situations.

CHAPTER 2

Early RAF Pilot Training

Born at home in a three-storey house in South Lambeth, London, I was the last of four children. My mother was the daughter of a small-time farmer in Shenley, Hertfordshire; my father, born in West Cowes, Isle of Wight, was very much into sailing, a very skilled carpenter and a good all-round DIY man. Despite his comparatively modest wage annual holidays were always spent away – usually in Cowes with relatives, especially during the main yacht-racing season, or with other relatives living in and around Sway in the New Forest. Walks down to Meade Ends, to gather some of the masses of bluebells and primroses still come easily to mind and also, most vividly imprinted on the memory, as a very small boy, standing on the fencing wires at the top of the cutting running down to Sway railway station, waving to the drivers and firemen of the steam trains pulling the great Bournemouth expresses down from Waterloo station in London. If they saw us they always waved back; at night, too, we watched them as they hurtled through the cutting, lit in the cab by the bright orange glow from the firebox.

My father was a dedicated yacht enthusiast and made the most magnificent scale models of the 6-metre racing yachts. These were some 7 ft long with an 8 ft high mast and a heavy leaden keel (moulded and poured at home in the utility room!). These were raced at the well patronised yacht club by the Rick pond – in the grounds of Hampton Court. With a strong wind blowing, catching and turning these fast moving models was a particular challenge; turning the nose round to head it off on to the other tack was normally all that was needed. The subsequent run downwind with spinnaker set was a riot of colour and wonderful to watch. If properly trimmed before release on the downwind leg the boat ran straight without coming ashore and made good time to the finish line.

Summer holidays in Cowes were inevitably based around sailing; the objects of much special attention were the huge 'J' class yachts – Endeavour, Britannia, Shamrock, Candida, Valsheda and the schooner Westward. When particularly strong winds were blowing the Westward would always appear way ahead of the others at the finishing line. The course was a complete circuit of the island starting with a gun fired from the Royal Yacht Squadron premises on the front. Once out of sight the entertaining antics of the sailors ashore from a visiting warship kept people amused – especially the struggles to climb the greasy pole and, occasionally, the wonderful sight of outgoing or incoming ocean liners from and to the Southampton docks from all parts of the world.

Other classes of yachts were much in evidence, sailing on courses well within visual range of the appreciative and mostly knowledgeable crowds along the sea front promenade. Leisure time in South Lambeth was put to good use, quickly attaining a fairly high standard of proficiency on roller skates and informal games of cricket and football (on nearby Clapham Common). Having successfully completed Primary School (St. John's Bowyer in Clapham) where one highly imaginative and dedicated teacher in particular (Mr. Pickford) stimulated and inculcated interest and competency in several subjects; reading Mark Twain's Tom Sawyer to us every Friday afternoon was particularly enjoyable and remembered. Winning a scholarship enabled me to follow my two older brothers to the Strand Secondary (Grammar) school, between Brixton and Streatham. Although often under a cloud with a dour and seemingly hostile Scottish housemaster (McMinn) I emerged from the shadows when it was learned that I could bowl a cricket ball far more accurately than most – with the result that McMinn's soon became the team to beat. Two 'hat-tricks' in away schools matches, and figures of 9 wickets for 17 runs, secured my place in the sun from then on.

The imminence of war saw us moved away from London en bloc and down into Surrey where we were allocated local families to live with. Soon after we were sitting the equivalent of 'O' levels at a school near Effingham, taking the bus daily from our digs in Great Bookham. Having rejoined my parents in their house near Wimbledon I took a job with a large power-station design and maintenance firm with a job in the drawing office. This was directed by a Mr. Ewbank, a huge impressive man who had been a pilot in the Royal Flying Corps, in France in the First World War, and who was naturally supportive of those of us enlisting to fly with the RAF. I immediately joined the local Air Training Corps and was immediately absorbed in all related flying subjects (aircraft recognition, engines, theory of flight, navigation, meteorology) and lots of marching and drill manoeuvres which, strangely perhaps, we thoroughly enjoyed.

But the RAF was waiting and hopes were high that I might at last get the chance to learn to fly. As we soon found out, this was to be under the new Empire Air Training scheme – with training aerodromes in Canada, America (as civilians – since the USA was not then at war), South Africa and Southern Rhodesia.

On the larger canvas... "arrangements had been made to transfer elementary and basic flying training to those areas within the Commonwealth least likely to come under direct enemy action. It was essential to keep the restricted air space over the British Isles clear of training aircraft and of course too many aerodromes could not be diverted from operational needs. Furthermore the close proximity of Britain to the Luftwaffe meant that a serious flying training programme was bound to become a target of some priority in the eyes of the German High Command: it would be all too easy for them to stop the flow of new pilots to the squadrons when the RAF would surely become paralysed. Then again there was the traditional British weather – hardly ideal for a non-stop training programme.

From these thoughts emerged the now famous Empire Training Scheme with its scores of elementary and service flying schools situated out of enemy reach.

Obviously the cost of transporting thousands of aircrew across the seas was high, both in terms of real money and, what was more important at the time, valuable shipping capacity. Then there was the attendant risk of sending thousands of the nation's above-average young men through U-boat infested waters – young men who had already assumed a degree of potential value for, prior to shipment they had already completed 6 months or so at one of the Initial Training Wings where a very thorough pre-flight training had been given them.

Pilot training during the war was based upon a policy of progressive elimination of all but the best candidates. Not unnaturally nearly everyone wanted to be a pilot, and during the early stages of the war the home flying schools were busy coping with the part-trained direct RAF entrants. However once the Empire Training Scheme got under way it was vitally necessary to have some arrangements which would prevent square pegs from getting into round holes; it is one thing to consider oneself a future bomber or fighter pilot but quite another matter when the training starts. Unlike peacetime club flying, these student pilots were put through a rapid and highly concentrated course, getting their wings after two hundred hours flying, when they would be expected to pilot some of the most complex equipment put into the hands of man at that time. No civil airline would consider placing a nineteen-year-old in command of a four-engined aircraft weighing the wrong side of thirty tons, sending him over Europe in hail, rain or snow with but a few hundred hours in his log book. Yet this fact is precisely what happened time and again, and the fact that the boys were generally able to cope is a true measure of the Empire Training Scheme.

To separate the square pegs from the round holes all candidates were accepted for aircrew under the classification PNB (Pilot/Navigator/Bomb Aimer). So labelled, the cadets went to ITW for comprehensive ground courses and on successful completion progressed to Grading Schools. Those considered below the average level of aptitude for pilot training continued their service in one of the other aircrew categories.

The Grading Schools were in reality pre-war, civil-operated Elementary Flying Training Schools, with one or two exceptions already equipped with Tiger Moths, so that the important task of categorizing all the war-trained aircrew for the RAF fell to the lot of the little biplane. It is because of its Grading School activities during this phase of the war that to fly a Tiger Moth became part of the experience of almost every RAF pilot". (Quoted verbatim from the book *The Tiger Moth Story* by Alan Bramson & Neville Birch, Airlife Publishing Ltd., Shrewsbury, England, 1964)

I officially volunteered to join on my 18th birthday and was placed on the reserve – since all flying schools, both at home and abroad, were full and there was a long waiting period. The initial examination was at Regents Park Aircrew Reception Centre where recruits were assessed and graded as suitable for training either as Pilot, Navigator or Bomb Aimer (PNB). There were lots of inoculations, more drilling, more lectures and in particular very stringent checks on health and co-ordination. For this latter one sat in front of a screen with cross wires marked on it; a white wandering light moved across the screen and one had to use the central control column and foot pedals to keep the light on the cross wires. Having successful negotiated these I was graded pilot and posted to an ITW (Initial Training Wing) unit based in the Toorak Hotel in Torquay. More marching, lectures and cross-country runs (across cold wet Devon fields with a glorious hot shower at the finish) kept us fighting fit. For dinghy drill the local open-air baths were used; these were filled with sea-water and were freezing cold and did nothing to encourage one to jump off the highest diving board to surface and climb into single and 4-man dinghies. With the final exams safely passed we foregathered to spend the evening in a special room at a local pub to celebrate our success.

A quick spot of home leave was followed by a posting to Elmdon RAF Grading School south-east of Birmingham where we were allocated to different flights to start the initial 12 hours or so of flying instruction on the immortal Tiger Moth biplanes. This was early January and to get the delicacy of feel for the feet on the rudder bar of this sensitive little plane, only shoes could be worn. The heavy fur-lined zipped flying boots were banned (although very glamorous and much desired) because, rightly, they blocked the sensitivity required for good rudder control. My instructor was Flying Office Hendy, a pleasant, kindly man and a magnificent pilot (as undoubtedly were all RAF instructors). At the end I happened one day to see his final remarks... "Rickman has good aptitude as a pilot and should go far". In fact just after the war's end I finished up in Hong Kong – although I hope that this was not what he meant!

One dark and dismal rainy morning we took off and climbed away up into the thick layers of strato-cumulus. As we broke through, out of this cloud layer, we emerged in to a 'winter wonderland' of bright sunshine – flying as if above a large sunlit snowfield broken only by occasional dark 'mountains' of cumulus. Magic indeed! "Time to start back for home – I've got her" came Hendy's voice over the intercom. I just had time for my "You've got her, Sir" when the plane was rolled over on to its back and I failed from then on to hear anything, My Sutton harness was clearly not tight enough to hold me and I slipped out smoothly until my waist was level with the top of the fuselage and the slipstream hitting me squarely in the face and preventing all speech; my fingers were locked firmly under the longerons. As I was about to part company with the plane and instructor, and doubtless descend upon some luckless suburban Birmingham family – in time for lunch (with luck) – the plane was righted quickly and I fell back into the cockpit again.

"Sorry old chap" came Hendy's voice over the intercom, "I always like to glide down inverted through these layer clouds. You didn't have your harness up tight enough – my fault – I should have warned you and checked before we took off". I flew the plane back much relieved and, crossing the Elmdon boundary fast at 30 ft, went in to make a smooth landing. "Well done – you should have no trouble with the final grading assessment – keep those landings straight and smooth – good luck". My final assessment was hurried because of time pressure but I made two 'daisy-cutter' [good quality bumpless] landings and given the green light to continue pilot training.

A quick spell of home leave was followed by what seemed a intolerable period of waiting to get to flying school and become front-line pilots (we hoped). Next came the first of many visits to the notorious Heaton Park Reception Centre. Situated just outside Manchester it received more than its fair share of rain and, with so many hundreds of RAF cadets forever marching about, the once glorious park quickly became a mud bath. We were housed in Nissan huts in each of which the central vertical iron stove took pride of place. It was kept fully stoked up and glowing red from top to bottom. Improvised 'Welsh Rarebits' pushed near to it, usually on the back of a metal shovel blade, were quickly sizzling merrily and in great demand to the 15 or so bored and still hungry residents.

To give us all a modicum of practical RAF experience we were posted to a variety of front-line aerodromes, where we performed various tasks from cookhouse washing up, toilet cleaning, vehicle washing in the Motor Transport section or minor office jobs (all to quench any feelings of superiority in we 'officer cadets'!). The first port of call for me was Stradishall – a major bomber station in Suffolk. This was equipped with the large but rather ungainly 4-engined Stirling and less-awkward-looking Halifax bombers. My job, helping in the stores, provided the valuable opportunity of fortnightly 'blanket' runs to a large laundry in London, with the chance of a couple of nights and some decent meals at home before racing back to catch the lorry to Stradishall. One rather solemn duty we cadets all shared was making up the funeral parties. With so many bombers coming back crippled and the crews badly shot up, even some planes with an unexploded bomb still hung-up in the bomb-bay, crashes were not too uncommon and our task was to march with the hearse and form the official firing party – shooting off volleys of blanks as a 'farewell' gestures to those recently departed this life.

This was followed by another visit to Heaton Park for what seemed like more pointless marching about, usually in the pouring rain, and cooking more tasty Welsh Rarebits on the back of a shovel. What seemed at the time to be merely an irritating waste of time was the continual calling of names to be answered and standing around in the huge theatre-like hangars. This tried the patience of most of the lads, all of whom wanted nothing more than to get to flying or navigation schools – mostly overseas. One Disciplinary-Sergeant on the stage and facing some 500-600 damp and bored aircrew cadets and hearing their murmurs of impatience and dissent, shouted belligerently "You useless shower of mummy's boys – you wouldn't say boo to a goose!". In the complete silence that followed there came a lone loud voice from the back – "Boo!". This resulted in immediate riotous laughter and the memorable picture of one red-faced and incoherent sergeant being coaxed off the stage by the officer-in-charge.

The next 'port of call' was Tempsford aerodrome near Bedford. This was used during the war both to train and to transport secret agents going into and being brought from isolated fields in occupied Europe. Arms, ammunition, explosives, medical dressings, food, torches, radio sets etc were all parachuted down in long steel containers. The agents, many of them young women, were landed in, or parachuted into, France or Holland from Lysander and the smaller Auster aeroplanes.

The next and last visit was to another heavy bomber station – this one at Upwood in Cambridgeshire – where Lancaster bombers and the new fast, all wooden de Havilland Mosquito aircraft were part of the famous Pathfinder Force. I was selected to work in the Wing-Commander's office – fetching the daily synoptic charts (weather forecasts) and keeping safe custody of the individual pilot's log books; several of which made very lurid reading! Wing-Commander Isen arranged for me to go on a pre-ops test flight in a Lancaster bomber. Flight Lieutenant Jackson and his crew were testing some new electronic and radar equipment that had been fitted. All had strange names – Oboe – Fishpond – H2S and it was only after the war that details of their development and the vital part they played in the air war against Germany became common knowledge.

As we flew out over the Wash I was sitting beside the navigator in a darkened section and although above a 10/10ths cloud cover, could see it quite clearly picked out in some detail by the rotating green strobe. I was called forward and asked to stand between the two pilots and to hold on tightly. I soon found out why. "Time for tea now – hold tight everyone" came the pilot's voice over the intercom a few seconds before he pulled the huge Lancaster bomber up sharply into a stall turn and let it fall sideways, the altimeter spinning furiously as we fell headlong down to earth. A smooth pull-out – a long gentle turn and we were lined up with the runway on which we touched down gently and rolled to a stop – masterly!

A quick delivery trip in a Mosquito came a day or so later – sitting behind the pilot (we needed no navigator for this short hop) with two huge propellers, the spinning tips seemingly only a foot or so from the plexiglas cockpit cover. Again a beautifully smooth landing – climbing out not without difficulty (one suspects that it would have been difficult to abandon this plane in a hurried emergency; although the aircrew flying it would be well practised in this important safety factor!). The trundle back was made in a noisy, and considerably slower Airspeed 'Oxford' communications plane.

But by now the wait for us was nearly over, and we were soon on our way back to Heaton Park for kitting out (tropical clothing). This consisted mainly of too-long shorts and the inevitable and quite ridiculous solar topee. "Looks like we're heading for Iceland" was one wag's comment. A couple of days later we moved to West Kirby where we received more inoculations and, to our surprise and delight, found ourselves under the care of the great Stanley (now deservedly Sir Stanley) Matthews – a shy, modest man with a quiet sense of humour and no regimentation at all. We all adored him and asked him lots of questions, as I'm sure did all of those others who had the good fortune to pass through his hands en route overseas. This was quickly followed by embarkation on to the huge (by our standards) RMS Andes which was to take us rapidly down to Cape Town – en route to our nominated flying schools.

My first introduction to the great African continent occurred early in January 1945 when, together with several hundred other would-be birdmen, we came ashore at Cape Town bound for an RAF Flying School in what was then Southern Rhodesia (now Zimbabwe). Three weeks or so earlier we had been coached from West Kirby to board the RMS. 'Andes' at Birkenhead. A little later, in the middle of the night, we left a very wet and windy Britain and headed out westwards via Liverpool Bay into the teeth of a very impressive north Atlantic storm. The 'Andes', a Royal Mail ship of some 30,000 tons, was capable of travelling unescorted at speeds up to 30 knots and thus able to avoid any German U-boats that may have been lying in wait. But despite her weight and speed the foam-capped hillsides of water, glinting glassy green, that gathered themselves together and rose up majestically in her path, lifted her bow with awesome ease and, as she passed over the crest and fell away into the trough behind, threw up her stern, causing her to shudder rhythmically as her propellers came close to the surface.

Our group was quartered at the back, in the basement, low-down aft – euphemistically known as 'steerage', where I was fortunate in opting for, and getting, a hammock. Few of us had ever tried sleeping in one of these before and we had to come to terms with the correct method of climbing in safely and staying in. For some, this initial baptism was bruising; though being mid-winter the warmth of their language was a welcome bonus! With a life-jacket for a pillow and a wooden spreader behind the head (both forbidden) I slept like a log. The regular surge and roll of the ship in the quartering seas provided a rocking motion to the hammock that was soporific.

Those who earlier had failed to come to terms with the enigmatic hammock, or who were unwise enough to opt for sleeping on the mess-deck tables, came sadly unstuck when, without warning and often in the middle of the night, the 'Andes' made several sudden changes of course at full speed – presumably zigzagging to avoid reported U-boat packs. This served to throw all the 'table-toppers' on top of those who, even more unwisely, had chosen to sleep on the floor! By this time many of the lads were sea-sick and next morning, with big seas still running, very few were able to appreciate the joke when a would-be comic in the purser's office played 'Someone's rocking my dream-boat' over the ship's PA system. Some of those who were destined for air navigation courses had been keeping a log of the ship's courses (with prismatic compasses) and approximate speeds. From this they calculated that we were nearing the coast of South America before we turned south-east to Freetown in Sierra Leone. (The Andes was probably avoiding U-boat packs).

The north Atlantic storms eventually gave way to completely calm windless weather as we approached and entered the doldrums, off the coast of West Africa. By now the ocean was a deep blue glassy carpet across which we glided at speed, sending up showers of flying fish, which shone for a few seconds in irridescent colours as they rose from the surface, sometimes gliding quite long distances before disappearing suddenly with a quick splash-down. Looking aft, the lines of the ship's wake stretched with mathematical precision out to the horizon on both sides. From time to time dolphins and porpoises picked up the ship's vibrations and came racing in to have some fun – leaping and plunging in and around the bow-wave, their bodies glistening in the sun as they rose from the surface and dived again and again, clearly having the time of their lives!

The 'Andes' docked in Cape Town early in January and we disembarked on to a waiting South African train for the 3-day journey up to Bulawayo and thence to our nominated flying schools. After passing through the beautiful and lush wine-growing areas of Paarl and Worcester the train began the long haul up the Hex River Valley into and through the Karoos – coming out finally on to the great central plateau, where the scenery gave way to open scrub-land, typical of much of the African uplands. Open observation platforms at the ends of the carriages gave ample opportunities to break the monotony of the endless cards games and reading and the chance to take in the passing scenery. At De Aar junction a 45-minute stop gave everyone the chance to invade the local shops. Fresh from the shortages of wartime Britain this was akin to releasing a plague of locusts into a well-stocked vegetable garden. In no time at all the place was denuded of drinks, gifts and clothes. Watches of course were in great demand, most of the lads choosing those with impressive sweep second hands, perhaps feeling that these gave the greater accuracy that would soon be needed by aspiring fighter and bomber pilots!

We reached Bulawayo in the middle of a spectacular tropical thunderstorm, with vivid 'trees' of pinkish-blue forked lightning arcing every few seconds followed immediately by deafening thunder-claps and with horizontal wind-driven rain that almost blotted out visibility. The issued gas capes gave us little protection and we were all soon soaked to the skin as we marched from the lorries to the reception centre. When we woke the following morning the sky was blue and cloudless and we revelled in the warmth of the sun. The next two weeks consisted of general familiarisation, with lectures on social behaviour (in a host country which, it was hoped, would stay friendly despite our presence) and on the risk of contracting some pretty horrible diseases prevalent in this part of Africa. Schistosomiasis (Bilharzia), a serious and debilitating disease caused by paired worms living in the liver and pelvic veins (for up to 30 years!) causing continuous internal bleeding and severe anaemia and caught by entering snail-infected water, was one such.

We were put through some practical field exercises aimed at giving us confidence in map-reading and in the use of the prismatic compass. Presumably this was so that we could find our way home again in the unlikely event (we hoped!) of a forced landing in the bush – away from the base airfield. For this, small groups were taken in a blacked-out lorry and put down some miles from a recognisable meeting point. This was marked on our map, as were the drop-off and collection points, and we were each given a map, compass, emergency rations and a full water bottle. The lorry quickly disappeared in a cloud of dust leaving us to work out the appropriate magnetic bearings, courses to steer, approximate distances and a rough Estimated Time of Arrival (ETA) for the rendezvous.

Walking in Indian file we set off across country, stopping every 15 minutes to check the bearing and allow the chap at the back, who had the map and was keeping us all on line, to change places. We passed a few African villages from which the children and dogs came running out to join in the fun and run and march alongside us. Having seen it all before the children would march proudly beside us, arms fully stretched while they shouted ‘Left – Right – Left – Right’ – making us all laugh at their accurate ‘pantomime’ approach. Our style was clearly more akin to that of the rural Africans’, most of whom think nothing of walking 20 or 30 miles to a market or meeting, usually at a comfortable gait and often either bare-footed or wearing motor-tyre ‘flip-flops’; in that heat we didn’t think much of it either! The dogs barked and the people waved and grinned – probably at our odd attire (khaki shirts, too-long shorts all topped with solar topees!). Apart from a few tick bites, the perpetrators of which were speedily removed when touched with a lighted cigarette end, and a little sunburn we had no other problems and eventually surprised ourselves and doubtless our instructors when, within 15 minutes of our ETA, we emerged from some fairly thick bush to find a tarmac road and the lorry within sight some 200 yards away.

We did three of these exercises, ranging in distance from 7 to 15 miles, and we enjoyed the challenge and the realisation that with careful navigation one need never be lost – merely have an undefined (probably wide) circle of uncertainty! The villagers were generally friendly and helpful and delighted when we shared our cigarettes with them; some even offered us food which, given the evident difficulties of growing it, we were reluctant to accept. During my subsequent 32 years in Africa, much of it working in 'bush' areas, I have had no reason to change these first impressions of the generous hospitality and friendliness of rural African communities.

After a few days exploring the delights of Bulawayo with its tree-lined streets, deliberately made wide enough to turn in with a span of oxen, we once again took the train up to Gwelo (now Gweru), mid-way between Bulawayo and Salisbury (now Harare). At Guinea Fowl we had our first look at the planes in which we would be training – the beautiful and shapely Fairchild Cornells with their 125 hp Ranger engines, flaps and sliding cockpit canopies – all painted a bright yellow and standing in smart lines waiting for us to climb in! These had superceded the Tiger Moths which, up until then, had done sterling service but which had suffered deterioration due to the dust and rough ground conditions. The Cornell, a low-wing monoplane, was very similar to the British 'Chipmunk'.

Guinea Fowl was an all-grass aerodrome a little under 5000 ft above sea level. Flying started at 06.00 hrs every morning, for calmer air and to avoid the afternoon turbulence, and since these early morning starts were very cold indeed we tended to drink our teas and coffees huddled round the huge urns put out on the tables. Flying was sometimes delayed while the thick frost was wiped off the wings and windscreens. Also we sometimes had to wait for the warmth of the sun to lift the 'guti' – a thick mist which precluded virtually all flying. Towards the end of the course we were flying in almost all conditions and became experts at spotting and avoiding the treacherous 'dust-devils' or miniature whirlwinds which could easily flip a small aeroplane upside down as you neared the boundary fence on final approach when landing.

My instructor was Flight-Sergeant Peter Pipe a huge, handsome, fair-haired rugby-playing (front-row forward) giant who, despite his size, handled the aeroplane with consummate delicacy and total mastery. After a few hours of the standard 'circuits and bumps' and glide-approach landings (with engine well throttled back) he climbed out shut his sliding hood and said “Off you go now laddie! Don’t bend it! Do me three nice circuits and landings and I’ll stand you a beer on your return!” With that he strode off without a backward glance.

I swing the plane round, head to wind, first check gyro compass on zero – unlock – adjust trim for solo – check 15 degree flaps – open throttle smoothly and column right forward to bring tail up. That’s better – now I can see where I’m going! Speed now 65 mph – column gently back and off we come. No feeling of nervousness, too much to think about. At about 500 ft slowly bring up flaps and at 700 ft ease the stick gently left into a smooth climbing turn still on full throttle, coming cross-wind at 1000 ft – throttle back for straight and level cruising – nice medium turn down wind – throttle back – let down 30 degrees of flap (stick forward a bit to balance) – final medium turn cross wind to line up with the airfield – check compass is on zero (dead into wind)- open canopy and lock back – cross boundary fence about 50 ft easing back on column – keep straight – now about 10-15 ft – throttle right back with column now fully back into stomach – all quiet now, sinking slowly – then the gentle rumble of all three wheels on the grass (a perfect ‘daisy-cutter!) – toes gently forward on the brakes – keep straight – stop – turn cross-wind to check no other aircraft are landing or taking off – raise flaps – turn and taxi back, swinging the nose from side to side for vision. First solo completed with a wonderful feeling of release and elation and – I’m on ‘Cloud 9’! Two more circuits and acceptably smooth landings later I taxied in, switched off and went into the flight hut to collect my winnings and slake my thirst!

This was followed by more continuous practice flying, sometimes dual but increasingly solo; there was strict emphasis on the basic manoeuvres such as stalling, spinning and the beautiful and graceful stall turns where the nose was pulled up high and, on the point of stall, the rudder bar was pressed firmly, left or right, and the plane slid sideways and downwards gathering speed rapidly in the dive until pulled up sharply again to repeat the process perhaps on the other side. Soon we were on to more advanced techniques – the slow roll being the most difficult. Instrument flying needed maximum concentration as did recovery from unusual positions – while under the hood, with only the instruments to guide you. Having put the plane into an almost impossible position, e.g. upside down – standing on one wing and at the point of stalling when the voice came over the intercom… “You’ve got her”. Fortunately, by this time, instrument reading was almost second nature and the recovery under the hood was immediate and fortunately correct! A very important lesson was to trust the instrument readings implicitly and not the 'seat-of-the-pants' impressions!

An instrument cross-country flight came next – again done entirely blind. Peter Pipe continued giving me courses to steer – any mistakes in instrument flying were made in complete silence – no corrections given. After a 3-legged flight lasting about an hour or more Peter Pipe's voice came "OK – you can come out now. See if you can recognise where we are"

I swung the nose left then gently again to the right and saw straight ahead Guinea Fowl aerodrome – and we were lined up for a straight run in; another hurdle successfully over.

For night flying the landing field was marked out with two lines of 'goose-neck' flares – large oil drums each with a long angled spout with a large flame burning from a wick at the end. These two rows of flares, about 20 yds between each pair could be clearly seen from the air. Judging the approach and landing between them from the air took practice but soon proved fairly straightforward. But for the first few night flights one's eyes never lost sight of that life-saving flare-path!

Low flying came next and this was clearly Peter Pipe's pride and joy. That he was a superb pilot was soon demonstrated as we approached the Kabanga bombing range, This was a large field about the size of two football pitches side by side and was covered with 10 ft high elephant grass. Kabanga was used at a later stage, to practice air-to-ground gunnery and bombing, when flying the faster Harvard aircraft from Thornhill aerodrome, some 10-15 miles from Guinea Fowl…

"I've got her" came his voice as we approached. Straight up into a steep turn on full throttle then over and down in a steep dive pulling out some 20 ft above the grass. Suddenly we went into a steep turn around the perimeter of the field but, by then, Peter Pipe had dropped us down so that the wing-tip was brushing the top of the elephant grass; he did a complete circuit of the field like this before straightening up and at about 20 ft above the ground flew between two adjacent trees and skidded around others until the trip culminated in a dive down into hippo Gorge – where he skimmed along the river almost touching the wheels on the backs of the group of somnolent hippos clustered together in a large pool.

On our way back to Guinea Fowl aerodrome he said "What's the betting that I can land this plane without hands on the control column?" To me this seemed impossible – "Very high odds against" I replied. I made a normal approach – checked and uncaged the gyro compass as we crossed over the signals area and came round on to the last cross-wind leg of the approach, "OK, I've got her" came his voice. He slid back the cockpit canopy and raised both hands on the sides of it. Mine hovered very close to the control column but didn't touch it. We crossed the downwind fence at some 30 ft and continued smoothly losing height, then the nose was gently raised a little. "Please cut the throttle" – I did so and almost immediately we touched down very gently in a 'tail-down wheeler' – no hands! "I won't take your money – I do it with my knees" he said over the intercom – as if this explained everything! What a man!

After some 30 or so hours of routine training procedures the time came to start night flying. Two or three trips with Peter Pipe were sufficient to convince me that flying at night was really no more difficult than in daylight – provided one could learn (surprisingly quickly!) not to lose sight of the life-saving flare-path and how to judge height and distance for the final approach and landing. This latter involved judging the correct angle of approach and the appearance of the two lines of flares – too low and they close up: too high and they open up.

When the time came for my being sent off for my first night-solo, the Sergeant pilot taking me for the pre-flight check, to save time, told me to go out and prepare everything whilst he filled in the appropriate authorisation forms. On reaching the plane, parked neatly enough, by the student who had just completed his night-flying session in it, from habit I began walking slowly round the plane to make the standard pre-flight checks – no flat tyres, the pitot-head cover removed etc and as I passed across the front of the plane I noticed a piece of wire dangling from the hub and a long split down both blades. When the instructor came out he understandably started berating me... "Why aren't you in the cockpit, strapped in, ready to start up and taxi out for a quick take-off?"

When I drew his attention to the cracked propeller he almost exploded. "Thank goodness you saw this; if you hadn't we would both have gone for the proverbial Burton. That prop would have disintegrated completely on take-off – not a very nice prospect. We'll scrub tonight's trip – you'd best go back to bed whilst I try to sort this out".

When the previous cadet pilot was roused from his slumbers and asked to explain what had happened, he said that he had completed his third solo flight and had noticed nothing unusual on his last landing – he had taxied in and parked as usual before going off to bed. Later, the subsequent examination of the downwind boundary fence showed clear signs of damage; the top two strands of wire had been broken and two pieces (still round the propeller hub) were missing. He had clearly made too low an approach, which he was lucky to survive, but how he didn't feel the jolt as he did so is difficult to explain... I was only thankful that the earlier routine pre-flight inspection training paid handsome dividends and that my 'on-duty' Guardian Angel was in good form! Two nights later the flight check was repeated and Peter Pipe sent me off to do 3 solo night circuits and bumps – all of which I did successfully and enjoyed. For ease of mind it doesn't pay to think back too much about what might have happened otherwise!

CHAPTER 3

More Advanced flying

Training at Thornhill – war and training cease – travels in the Far East – mountaineering in Norway.

Having successfully completed the Elementary Flying Training Course (EFTS) the next move was to No. 22 Service Flying Training School at Thornhill on the other side of Gwelo. My new instructor was Sgt. Mitchell from Eastbourne. Thornhill was bigger, had tarmac runways and was equipped with the more powerful and manoeuvrable Harvard low-wing monoplanes, with retractable undercarriage and 550 hp radial Pratt & Witney Wasp engines. One initially surprising feature was the comparative violence of the machine when going into a spin. One moment with the control column held back and the throttle closed all was quiet and calm; the next one wing had seemingly been wrenched down by some giant hand, the plane had turned almost on to its back and the earth below was spinning round in a general blur. "That's fine", said the instructor's calm voice over the intercom, "Now, control column right forward and hard opposite rudder – like this" – and within a couple of seconds the earth below had sobered up and stopped spinning crazily and I felt the 'g' force as we pulled steadily out of the dive. "All very straight-forward – you'll soon get the hang of it" came his voice in my ears, "Your turn now – let's try a spin to the left – you've got her". Two or three spins later and all was well – it was straightforward – no problem. The Harvard was a beautifully responsive aeroplane with no serious vices. (P1.1)

All in all RAF flying training was totally absorbing, sometimes scarey but mostly quite exhilarating and exposed us to many new challenging and exciting experiences. It gave us confidence in our own abilities; though this was sometimes misplaced in some who came back with festoons of green water-weed, from a nearby lake, adorning the wheels and the luckless student who, when making a night landing approach to Thornhill, lined up on the row of lights at the local Gwelo railway marshalling-yard, instead of the row of goose-neck flares down the runway. He realised his mistake when he saw himself flying alongside rows of carriages and trucks before making an immaculate (presence of mind) wheels-up landing just before entering a small wood; this clipped his wings a little (both literally and metaphorically) but he climbed out with only minor cuts and bruises.

Yet another one earlier, who rode his luck mercilessly, was a cheerful lad called Bates who, returning to Guinea Fowl from lengthy high-altitude aerobatics practice, throttled back for the long steep gliding turns to reduce height – completely forgetting to rev up his engine every 500 ft to clear the oil from the plugs. When at some 2000 ft he opened the throttle to level out before joining the circuit there was no response from the engine. Since he was still on the wrong side of the rocky Selondi Range, with only rock-strewn shrub beneath him, he was immediately aware of having to make the decision to bale out and parachute down or try the almost impossible task of making a forced landing. Fortunately his guardian angel was on overtime and, when all seemed lost, the engine gave one or two coughs and started up again. Another luckless soul flying with us at Guinea Fowl, was Jimmy H. On his first solo cross-country from Gwelo to Bulawayo (and back), he temporarily forgot the safety instructions given us at briefing… 'that for the first part of the outward leg, flying south-west, the railway is away on the starboard side and, if you lose sight of it, you steer a little to the right until you find it, then follow it down to the airfield at Induna – just before reaching Bulawayo station'. Unfortunately, while enjoying the first few heady minutes of flying solo away from the aerodrome (probably dog-fighting with his mates – a common practice!), he crossed the railway without noticing it. Shortly after, unable to see it and with no other planes in sight, he turned right and headed out over largely uninhabited open bush country – across the Shangani river. Before finally running out of petrol he saw some native huts ahead but failed to reach them – landing instead in a field of 10ft high elephant grass. With intelligent use of the screw cap on the upper landing light as a container, he transferred enough remaining fuel from his spare tank to make another take-off, blind, through this grass. That he made it into the air was a major achievement but alas it was short lived. The engine cut again at about 400 ft up but his second landing brought him within sight of some local herdsmen who, by sign language, offered to help. They guided him to what turned out to be a Mission Station some 45 miles away. Having covered this distance with hardly a stop he arrived there totally exhausted and was put to bed and re-hydrated. The missionaries reported his safe arrival by radio to

Guinea Fowl and, next day, the Chief Flying Instructor flew out and landed in a nearby field that had been cleared of termite hills by Mission staff. Jimmy was praised for organising this, for lighting a small smoke-fire to indicate wind direction for landing and for his presence of mind in emergency.

All flying training ceased with the end of the war; only those very few willing to sign on in the permanent RAF were able to continue to get their 'wings'. In our group only one did so – my room-mate a young regular RAF cadet. The last I heard of Stan he had his wings and was a Flight Lieutenant pilot.

The voyage home in the new Mauretania was pleasant enough though the Bay of Biscay bared its teeth and gave us an unpleasant reminder of its power and notoriety – the bow waves sending spray over half way up the mast. Since I still had some two years to serve before my demob was due, and with further flying now out of the question, I chose to attend a course as a Motor Mechanic – the most useful of the options on offer. After a 3-month course at Melksham, where the high points were to assemble a small truck and put together a complete working differential gear-box – a brilliant piece of engineering design which allow the rear wheels to move at different speeds as e.g. when cornering, while maintaining a positive drive to both.

With the course successfully completed I was posted overseas again – this time to join a unit in Calcutta. A long and cold flight in a Liberator with short stops at Istres (Marseilles), Castel Benito (Libya) – Shaiba (Basra) and Delhi we finally landed at Dum Dum airport Calcutta only to find on arrival that the unit was in the midst of packing up for a move down to Rangoon. Once everything was loaded on to the comparatively small coastwise steamer, the S.S. Salween, we set sail in the late afternoon. Those of us opting to sleep in a hammock were told not to hang them in the mess deck until after the evening meal. One individual, more prescient than the rest of us, had noticed one hammock position immediately beside an open port-hole to which a large metal air scoop had been fastened. He took the chance and slung his hammock right beside it. I strung mine in the centre of the mess deck immediately opposite a wide companionway leading to and from the upper deck.

I was woken in the very small hours by my hammock banging against the mess-deck roof on both sides – to the almost continuous crashing of thunder. I opened my eyes to two truly memorable sights: one was the sea pouring in through our friend's porthole, via the air-scoop and filling his hammock; the other was a constant stream of blankets and their owners who had rather unwisely opted to sleep on the open deck. Fortunately no-one was lost overboard which was something of a miracle seeing that, with no warning, we had sailed slap into the middle of a tropical cyclone in the Bay of Bengal. We disembarked finally at Rangoon and immediately moved up country to a former Japanese airstrip cut out of the jungle at Hmawbi some 35 miles from Rangoon. The cinema consisted of rows of empty oil drums for seats and the screen a large whitish bedsheet strung between the trees. The film was changed every Saturday. Fortunately our stay there was short and we were soon on our way again – this time to Hong Kong, with short stops en route at Singapore and Saigon.

Finally a young Scottish driver and I were posted back to Calcutta – this time to join the RAF Police in their huge house at Ballygunge. For this trip we were aboard the S.S. Aronda which we shared with a large crowd of Indian 'Other Ranks' being repatriated.

In Cacutta, unfortunately, this was the time of the break-up of the Indian sub-continental populations and was exemplified by the horrifying Hindu-Muslim riots. We had to take several people to hospital who had been either stabbed or badly burned by the suphuric acid – thrown in open bottles. This acid was stolen from the nearby jute-processing factories on the outskirts of Calcutta; the local trams and buses were fitted with wire-gauzed windows and carried large bottles of saline with huge wads of cotton wool, since they were common targets. The riots themselves were frightening and at one time there were many dead bodies lying in the streets sometimes for days. On several occasions escaping groups came to our gate pleading for admittance and sanctuary from the gangs chasing them not far behind. But sadly, this was not possible since we had been ordered to keep well clear of the fighting and to take no sides in this religious dispute.

I managed a quick 2-week spot of leave and took the train from Sealdah station in Calcutta to Siliguri where we changed on to what was almost a toy train – to take us up the steep and twisting track to Darjeeling. During this latter trip, on several occasions one of the driver's mates would jump down and run alongside the engine throwing handfuls of sand under the wheels. In Darjeeling we were able to sample what for me was the Prince of Teas – 'Flowery Orange Pekoe'. But the clearest memory came on the second evening when the convection currents in the nearby valley finally lifted the dense mist that had hidden the mountains since our arrival. The unveiling of this magnificent and beautifully snow-covered mighty Himalayan range of mountains – 36 miles away but still hugely filling the sky, with the mighty Kangchengjunga (third highest peak in the world) proudly aloof with its massive skirts of snow and ice, and tumbling glaciers was a picture never to be forgotten. Early next morning we made a short journey to Tiger Hill where we caught a quick glimpse of the summit of Everest some 70-80 miles away.

Time for demob was approaching and was soon translated into a long and boring train journey made noticeable by the total lack of water, for drinking or washing, and by the sudden halt at a small station in the wee small hours when a reputedly Hindu-Moslem fight broke out and several people were knifed and severely injured. From Delhi we were quickly routed out to the reception centre at Deolali (which, for some, still retains overtones of mental stress!). A few more days waiting then finally boarding the 'boat home' – the twin-funnelled 'Arundel Castle' – for the trip back to 'Blighty' via the Suez. This was a voyage memorable for the massively attended impromptu sing-songs on the foredeck, where I played guitar together with a number of other amateur musicians, travelling across the Indian Ocean on a warm balmy evening under a magificent star-studded southern firmanent and the amazingly beautiful noctilucent flourescence in the sea at night. I took advantage of an offer to leave the boat temporarily at Port Suez and visit the museum of antiquities in Cairo, before joining it again at Port Said. The it was back to rainy dismal Liverpool – a train to London – swapping a solar topi for a trilby hat – a new civvy suit – and freedom!

It was when I first joined the Air Training Corps (ATC) in Merton, prior to applying to join the RAF, that I first met Len (Leonard Burchell); he was the Flight Sergeant of our group and we quickly became firm friends. We shared a sense of the ridiculous and a great love for music – classical, swing and jazz. In 1942 we joined the RAF together for pilot training but he unfortunately failed a critical eye examination and opted for a service career in radar. He spent much of the war years in the Outer Hebrides manning the radar defence chain. After the war he joined the International Oil Consortium in Abadan and prospered as an accountant, making many friends and learning to speak some Persian. In Abadan he met and married Mary, previously a ward sister at St. Bartholomew's Hospital in London, who had moved to a hospital in Abadan. By the time he left Persia he was the Financial Director, based in Tehran. Soon after he joined British Petroleum becoming Managing Director (Chemicals) before finally retiring to settle in Johannesburg, he and Mary choosing to live out their lives among the many friends that they had made there.

Our other friend was Peter Hughan who worked in a London office and soon after the war's end joined us firstly in hill-walking, in the English Lake District, and later when we went mountain walking in Norway. Our paths parted temporarily when Len went off to Abadan and I went to work in Kenya. Pete accepted a transfer to Zimbabwe where he met and married Jean in Bulawayo. Later, with their two sons they moved up to a house on the outskirts of Harare where they still remain, reluctant to leave the country they love while waiting for better times. Len, sadly now a widower, heads a major charity near Jo'burg helping to run a home for those severely handicapped and disabled – of all colours and creeds… Happily, we three still manage to keep in touch.

Before dispersing overseas we decided to spend some time together walking in the Jotunheimen district (aptly named: Home of the Giants) in central Norway. Using Len's Fiat 500 Topolino car (with its fold-down roof) we loaded up the tent, ice axes, climbing rope, crampons, boots and sleeping bags – drove up to Newcastle and boarded the Fred Olsen steamer bound for Bergen. Once ashore we drove through some truly wonderful scenery culminating in the precipitous descent into Gudvangen.The next stage was a smaller fjord-water-bus which sailed through the dark waters between vertical rock walls to join the great Sognefjord which ramifies into the very heart of the Jotunheimen and links up all the villages and hamlets en route. Leaving the ferry at Scholden we reclaimed the car, drove through rugged rock-strewn scenery to Tutagrö and eventually reached Elveseter. Here we unpacked and spent one night in glorious self-indulgent luxury. Next morning, shouldering our now weighty rucksacks we started along the winding track – ever upward – to Juvasshütte.

'What the Lake District means to the British and the Yosemite Valley to the Americans, that is what the Jotunheimen means to the Norwegians' – an enormous expanse of mountains, glaciers, highlands, lakes and waterfalls – with a series of well-equipped mountain lodges connected by trails that are clearly marked by stone cairns (vordet). The rocks are old (Pre-Cambrian) and consist mainly of wonderful gabbro – safe and perfect for climbing.

The Juvasshütte was a large hostel and well attended. Next morning we joined a group of Norwegian and Swedish youngsters and two elderly (but still very active) Afro-Americans to climb to the summit of Galhöpiggen – at 2469 m. the highest mountain in Norway. Half-way across the ice-field we roped-up to cross some rather large lateral crevasses which also obstructed the final route up to the summit. I had borrowed a guitar from the hostel so we were able to have an enjoyable sing-song all sitting on and around the summit cairn. The wind-blown snow finally drove us to seek shelter in the wooden hut on the summit. The descent, again roped up for the first mile, was pleasant and leisurely in glorious sunshine – all singing mostly Scandinavian songs interspersed with such favourites as 'My bonnie lies over the ocean', 'John Brown's body' and 'Green grow the rushes oh' etc.

The next day, accompanied by a few of our new friends we took the trail across the glacier to Spiterstulen hostel. The hostel is an old saeter [Norwegian Summer farm in the mountains] owned by Eiliv Sulheim. It is huge and surrounded by snow-capped mountains and glaciers; it also has a huge sloping access door in the roof so that, in winter, travellers can still find shelter when the saeter is snowed under. We pitched our tent by the river and were soon joined by Eiliv himself. The news of our playing and singing on the summit had reached him and he had come to ask if I would like to join him in playing for dancing in the evening after dinner. Eiliv was a certified mountain guide and, at that time, held the record for the fastest ski run down from the summit of Galdhöpiggen – at an average speed of 70 mph! He also played the piano accordian with equal competence (but not so fast) and had a seemingly endless list of songs and dances.

In the basement was a large wooden-floored dance hall with a small stage at one end. When we started to play the floor was quickly filled with swirling and singing couples – many in highly coloured sweaters and all dancing in their socks. During the evening we were joined by a young English geologist, Geoffrey Brazier, who was studying glaciology at Cambridge University for a PhD degree. He was in the middle of boring holes down into the glacier ice to count and measure the many different varved clays that mark the chronology of the retreat of the Svellnosbre glacier during the last European ice sheet.

We spent a fascinating day with him climbing all over the Svellnosbreen, exploring the ice caves and the maze of crevasses (Pl.2) The following day we decided to move on – by making the first spring crossing of the long Hellstyggebre glacier a huge humped-back mass of ice flowing between two quite high mountain ridges. Three Norwegians and two Swedish lads decided to come with us. Our 150 ft climbing rope was adequate so we agreed. Once roped-up and in line we climbed up the glacier tongue on to the snow-covered surface. Transverse crevasses were plentiful and slowed us up since the leader had first to see the slight hollowing of the snow, then prod with the ice-axe to test the depth and whether it was safe or narrow enough to walk or jump across. We did this all on a tight rope; if the leader failed to see the snow-covered crack and broke through the snow covering into it, the person behind would immediately lean back hard; this stopped the leader going in too deeply and he was easily able to extricate himself… At the top, before starting the descent of the other half, we found ourselves facing a major thunderstorm sweeping up across the glacier between the two ridges, coming straight at us.

The sky ahead was very black, the lightning was continuous and the thunder becoming louder and it was clear we had to find shelter quickly. Coming to a large rock at the side of the glacier we quickly rammed the ice axes into the snow some small distance away then all jumped down into the hollow, which the wind-driven snow had formed around it, and huddled together to await the passing of the tempest. Pass it did, but not before frightening us all half to death with the incessant lightning, deafening crashes of thunder and the sight of static electricity dancing round the heads of our ice axes only a few yards away. Eventually the sun came out again and the receding grumbles of thunder faded as we made good progress down the far side.

Coming off the glacier one last surpise awaited us; although we could see the Gjendebu hostel only some 300 yards away, to reach it we first had to wade across a wide, fast-flowing river fed with melt-water. One at a time and still roped for safety we waded through the freezing water, unroped and ran the final stretch into the warm and sheltering hostel. We had a hot shower – hung our clothes to dry in the warm boiler room and went into the lounge to work our way through the drinks and dinner menus!

Near the end of our Jotunheimen tour next day we did the easier 5 hour trek back to Spiterstulen for more singing and dancing and, next day to do some more snow and ice climbing on the Svellnosbre glacier. Again we had some of our friends with us including the two Swedish lads. Well roped up we climbed over the crevasses and into many of the wonderful ice caves – some of them so narrow and sited over a crevasse that to enter one had carefully to creep along with one foot on either side of the dark blue gap below! But the views of them and those from within them were wonderful and well worth the effort.

Next morning we sadly took our leave of our many friends at Spiterstulen, took advantage of a Landrover to take us back to Elveseter, where we wallowed in a hot bath, had a huge meal and a good night's sleep before packing the wee Fiat and driving our way out, via Flåm, Stryn and Olden where we boarded a coast-wise steamer for the journey back to Bergen. A quick visit to the old Hanseatic League buildings along the quay side, then a trip up the Fløyen funicular railway for a magnificent view out across the city of Bergen and the coastline and so back to the Fred Olsen steamer for a rather choppy crossing of the North Sea to Newcastle and so home.

CHAPTER 4

A Radical Change of Direction

From Mapping to Medical Research

Prior to my arrival at the Aircrew Reception Centre in Regents Park, London, in 1943, as mentioned earlier, I had been a trainee draughtsman with Ewbank & Partners, a small but influential firm of power-station consultant engineers. When I returned after the war, the firm had moved to an office near Hyde Park Corner in central London. This involved daily rush-hour commuting – a pleasure to be avoided, as most of those who suffer it daily will readily testify. All members of the Ewbank staff were kind and understanding and did everything possible to help me acclimatise to civilian life. I stuck it manfully for a few months but, one morning, having been standing in considerable physical and mental discomfort in a smoke-filled compartment of a toilet-less train, held at signals for 20 minutes outside Victoria Station, I finally decided that, whatever the future might hold, if I was to retain any spark of sanity, changes of location and vocation had become imperative.

I gave in my notice and soon joined the ranks of the 'maniacs and misfits' who then constituted the bulk of the new recruits to H.M. Ordnance Survey – a heterogeneous collection of interesting, intelligent, mostly likeable ex-service personnel. They included former commandos, tank drivers, RAF aircrew, marines, submariners, even secret agents, all shunning the conventional 9 to 5 office routine – choosing instead the outdoor life afforded by practical field cartography. Large-scale mapping is a challenging and fascinating occupation. Every day was full of incident, visiting new places in all weathers, meeting many people, working on the roof of a hospital one week and possibly in a railway marshalling yard, brewery or factory the next. However, once transferred to the plotting and traverse computations section at Chessington, the scene changed abruptly – and not for the better. Working with the continual clatter of a double-bank Brunsviga mechanical calculating machines (long since replaced by silent computers) in the company of 20-30 others, became for me reminiscent of Charlie Chaplin in '*Modern Times*' – the twitching hands continuing the mindless flicking of the metal levers and handle, backwards and forwards, long after the day's stint was finished. The noise was horrendous and, for me, not to be tolerated for much longer. Another change was clearly indicated!

One fateful day, as it turned out to be, whilst shopping in the nearby town on my way home, I sought temporary shelter from a providential shower of rain in a small second-hand book-shop. While browsing there my attention was caught by the title of a seemingly insignificant little book – "*Shadows in the Sun*" (by Stephen Taylor & Phyllis Gadsden). Flicking through the pages I was immediately impressed by the beautifully coloured diagrams and attractive disease distribution maps and, strangely perhaps, by the subject matter – tropical diseases. Many of us are fascinated by maps; even at school I loved nothing better than to draw them during geography lessons – all in full colour, with blue for the seas, lakes and rivers, browns and greens for the hills and lowlands, red and black dots for the major towns and villages; with a few lines of latitude and longitude to add a touch of verisimilitude! This lovely little book, with its clear diagrams, maps, pictures and concise informative text, was irresistible; but as I bought it and took it home to read, I little realised just how fundamentally it was to change my life.

The life cycles and distribution of the parasites and vectors of malaria, river blindness, sleeping sickness, elephantiasis, leprosy and others were set out; also, something of the history of each disease was caught with thumb-nail sketches of the work of the early pioneers, recent advances in research, diagnosis and treatment and an outline of the residual problems preventing proper control or eradication. Particularly evocative to me was the graphic description of the famous 'Anchau Experiment' (by Dr. 'Tam' Nash). Anchau, a village on a cattle route near Zaria in northern Nigeria, had been progressively invaded by the surrounding bush. When this later became infested with the rapidly spreading woodland-savannah tsetse flies (*Glossina morsitans*), the numbers of sleeping sickness cases rose alarmingly, with one third of the total population becoming infected. How the people were resettled into a newly constructed tsetse-free village called 'Takalafia' (Hausa: 'walk in health') is an inspiring story. Old Anchau village, by then totally engulfed by the tsetse-infested bush, was eventually pulled down and totally abandoned. Pictures of an elderly emaciated African sitting on the ground with one hand to his head, an advanced sleeping sickness case (with parasites in the cerebral-spinal fluid surrounding the brain and spinal cord) remains with me to this day – even though I have now seen very many such cases at first hand – in the villages of east and central Africa.

Reading this little book served to reawaken a long-buried interest in biological sciences and stimulated an active reappraisal of my future plans. I was now 32 years of age with little or no idea of where I was going or what I was going to do when I got there. Now, thanks to this little book, there was a glimmer of hope – but the 'careers bus' was already about to pull away so, if I was to travel with it, there was no time to lose – I must climb aboard. At best I would have yet another 'stand-up' seat; at worst I would find that, as with many others, 'there is a tide in the affairs of man which, taken at the flood, leads on to disaster' – probably with the bus once again heading in the wrong direction! The decision as to my future was now clear. I mentally spun a double-headed coin, called 'Tails' (out of sheer defiance) and immediately set about looking for a job as a 'Trainee Medical Adviser to the Third World'.

'Lady Luck', aghast at such presumption, nevertheless relented sufficiently to bring to my notice an advert in a daily paper for a Junior Locust Control Officer (Southern Sudan & Ethiopia) put there by that beneficent body, H.M. Crown Agents for the Colonies, Millbank, London. I quickly slipped my application into the post and waited for the Agents of the Crown to beat a path to my door. I had a long time to wait. In their own good time, several sobering weeks later, I received the official envelope containing an invitation to attend for interview in one of the many cells of the Millbank honeycomb.

There were 3 interviewers – one an adminstrator (as I supposed him to be), the second a UK-based scientist (as it later transpired) and the third was a well-built man with very fair hair and a swarthy complexion, who had clearly spent much of his life in sunnier climes. The administrator opened the bowling... "Mr. Rickman?" I nodded and managed a weak smile, "Please sit down". Never one to argue in the face of superior odds I duly collapsed in what I hoped was a reasonably tidy heap. I was very nervous. My education, interests and lack of any special knowledge or qualifications were quickly laid bare. He went on...

"Now perhaps you'd be kind enough to tell us, in your own words, why (he very kindly omitted 'on earth') you want to join the Desert Locust Control Service?" Since entering the room I had been asking myself the same question. Honesty was clearly the order of the day – but I had one trump card: I played it now. "To be truthful – I don't" I replied.

If this surprised them, they hid it well – probably being well used to candidate eccentricities. The administrator raised a questioning eyebrow "This is interesting – then would you mind telling us why you have applied for this post?" – the obvious corollary... "and why you have wasted our valuable time and the Crown Agent's money" was courteously suppressed. "To be honest", I said, "I would much rather work in a sleeping sickness control programme; it is my hope that, were I fortunate enough to be chosen for this post (I added hurriedly, hedging my bets), once in Africa it might be easier to transfer from locust to tsetse work".

"How much do you know about sleeping sickness?" – this was the scientist, smiling slightly "perhaps even its scientific name?". My avid reading now paid dividends and my practice with the word trypanosomiasis allowed it to slip easily off the tongue. I followed this with a fairly succinct summary of sleeping sickness – memorised from 'Shadows in the Sun'. Even I was impressed. 'Dr. Suntan' now came on to bowl .

"Mr. Rickman, I see from your CV that you have already visited Africa, during your service with the RAF". I nodded. "How did you like it?" he asked with a smile. I met that in the middle of the bat. "Very much", I said, "It's very big and colourful and I liked the climate very much". As a timely and truthful afterthought I added... "I also liked what little I saw of the African people. That's part of my reason for wanting to work there".

Then he bowled me a 'bouncer'... "Do you know how to use an oil-immersion microscope?" he asked, affably enough. This floored me completely; I had never even heard of it. "To be frank", I said, "I don't even know what it is but I am sure that I could soon learn to do so". I was mentally back on my feet again – shaken but with my wicket still intact. He then bowled me the googly... "Yes, that may be so, but an important part of your service abroad would be to train African staff. At the moment they would have to train you". Clean bowled! He smiled sympathetically as my spirits tried to get up off the floor.

After giving me a brief but clear overview of the nature of Desert Locust Survey and Control work, I was asked to wait outside for a few minutes while they conferred. Five minutes later I was called back in and invited to take a seat. The administrator then looked up from his notes and said... "My colleagues and I are convinced of your interest and desire to work in disease control in Africa, However, we feel that you would be wise to gain more scientific training and knowledge before doing so – perhaps obtain some qualification, even a degree? It's not too late" he added confidingly, with an encouraging smile; he went on..."In that way you would considerably enhance your value to those you wish to serve, and thus your own chances of success". If any of those wise and kindly men read this and remember, I hope they will accept my sincere thanks for their sound advice; for me, at least, it paid handsome dividends.

I travelled home deflated but with a spark of hope still burning. At least I had taken the first step – now for the second. Within a week I had signed on for evening classes in 3 'A' level science subjects – Zoology, Botany and Geology. A fortnight later I received confirmation from the Crown Agents that I had in fact been selected for the Desert Locust Control post. In my letter declining their offer, I thanked them for the sound advice given me at the interview, which I was now taking; and I promised to contact them again when I had successfully completed my present studies; but I doubt this raised their expectations much!

Evening classes soon became a way of life and a pleasant contrast to the clatter of the calculating machines in the survey traverse computations room. I slipped easily into the 'more mature student' role. The standard of teaching at the Kingston Technical College (now a University) was very high and the atmosphere friendly but purposeful. Lee Tanfield, the excellent lecturer in Zoology, was a highly intelligent and very attractive young lady with a very lively sense of humour. Geology field trips to the Long Mynd in Shropshire and to the Girvan coast in Ayrshire were a delight – full of interest and good humour. As luck would have it I had only recently returned from exploring and climbing among the mountains and glaciers of central Norway just before the A-level exams. I had a major geology question on glaciers for which I wrote 14 pages with many detailed diagrams; this gained me a mark of distinction – lucky again! Some time earlier, whilst working on the large-scale resurvey of the Epsom region, I went into a private school (New Sherwood) to seek permission from the headmaster to map the school and grounds. He was a tall dark-haired bearded man and greeted me warmly. When I explained the purpose of my visit, he asked if I would help him demonstrate the practical proof of the Pythagoras theorem. No problem! With the students gathering the pegs to stick into the ground we quickly taped out a large right-angled triangle and the squares on the three sides.

Little did I realise then that, much later, I would repeat this practical demonstration under very different circumstances!

John Wood, the Headmaster, was a Scottish classics graduate from Glasgow University, an ex RAF Flying Officer and a born mountaineer. We became firm friends and with Aubrey Dunn, the young and dynamic science teacher, we did many climbs together, in winter and summer, mostly in Glencoe, Glen Nevis and on the Cobbler at Arrocher. One of the parents whose son was at the school was Dr. 'Bill' Bray who was then studying the development cycle of the malaria parasite at the London School of Hygiene & Tropical Medicine – working under Professor Garnham, a world-famous malariologist. At that time Bill was looking for staff to work with him in a new malaria project planned for northern Liberia and, learning of my interest in tropical diseases and my course of studies, now nearly completed, asked if I would like to join his team.

Unfortunately, soon afterwards, the nature and scope of this new project was radically changed and precluded the recruitment, at that time, of any new staff. Before he left for West Africa, Bill Bray suggested I might like to visit the medical parasitology laboratories at the 'London School' and, whilst there, meet another medical scientist, a Dr. Ronald Heisch, who was home on leave from Kenya and, happily for me, also looking for new staff to work with his team at the Medical Research Laboratories in Nairobi. Dr. Heisch, a quite remarkable man, was the Director for many years of a small but very dynamic and deservedly renowned medical research unit, the Division of Insect-Borne Diseases (DIBD) situated next to the large Jomo Kenyatta Hospital. Dr. Heisch had been deputy to Professor Garnham but had assumed command when he accepted the chair in Medical Protozoology at the London School.

Ronald Heisch was slight of build, sharp featured, with thin sensitive fingers and a well-modulated voice. When I first met him in Prof. Garnham's office at the 'School' he handed me two small, green female figurines, probably jade, saying "What do you think of these – aren't they beautiful". I agreed – they were. The professor's eyes twinkled behind his glasses and in his high-pitched voice said... "Ronnie, whilst Mr. Rickman may well be interested in female figures I'm sure that, just now, he would rather like to know something of the work of the DIBD – and what he would be doing there – assuming that he is able and willing to join you" he added with a conspiratorial smile. They were old friends and shared, among other things, a deep love of music; both were talented performers.

Carefully replacing the two figurines in their wrappings Dr. Heisch went on... "Well, Rickman, you seem to be the kind of chap we're looking for; I'm sure that you will fit in well. The work is very varied and involves travelling and working in different parts of Kenya. The post will be that of junior Entomological Field Officer". It all sounded too good to be true, but there was even better to come... "We are a small friendly group but very active and you will find the country very interesting. There will be plenty of opportunity for you to continue your studies; in fact we'll get you a Government bursary to help you complete your science degree". This was really excellent news. He went on. "The post will have to be advertised of course, but I am sure you will have a very good chance of being selected, provided you wish to join us".

Ronnie Heisch was a strange mixture – a brilliantly gifted Cambridge University medical graduate he had a natural flair for research and was very much his own man. Soon after his arrival in Kenya, fairly or unfairly he had acquired the reputation of being an 'enfant terrible'. To keep him quiet and out of harm's way, he had been posted to Wajir in the very hot and arid desert of the North-East Frontier Province. This plan backfired, however, for news soon began to filter back to Medical H.Qs in Nairobi of the wonderful work that he was doing there, in particular his successful operations, many of them carried out by light of hurricane lamp, and his lengthy and frequent tours of his fiefdom on the back of a camel – dispensing medical care to even more remote village communities and settlements. Most of these never saw a doctor from one year's end to the next. Instead of being 'out of sight-out of mind' as had been hoped, Dr. Heisch had by now become something of a celebrity.

Later, when telling of these earlier days, he recalled that there had been one local chief who was determined to give him a hard time – by making regular and extravagant demands upon his time and energy for what were mostly bogus complaints. On one such occasion, having been called yet again by the chief, to come quickly on an urgent matter, he made the long and uncomfortable journey, by camel and in the heat of the day, only to find the chief complaining of mild constipation. To teach him a lesson he administered what he called a 'liberal dose of phenolphthalein aperient'. As he remarked later... "it rather restricts the amount of trouble you can cause anyone, Rickman, when you're having 40 motions a day!". But the chief had the last laugh. He sent a runner a few days later with a note to say that, due to his wonderful treatment, he had never felt fitter in his life! Thereafter they were firm friends – the chief tacitly acknowledging that he had met his match.

The second interview with H.M. Crown Agents for the Colonies was a far less daunting experience, although the questions were searching enough. My hopes rose considerably when, as I was leaving, the chief interviewer smiled and said... "You should receive the official notification, as to whether or not you have been selected for this post, within the next two weeks. But I'm sure that you will enjoy working in Kenya. Good luck!" Confimation duly arrived together with a cheque for kitting out. I was booked to sail on the S.S. Warwick Castle leaving London for Mombasa in mid-January 1956.

I approached Professor Garnham again, this time to ask if I might spend the remaining three months working in his department, on a voluntary basis, to learn a little tropical parasitology and some basic laboratory techniques and procedures. This turned out to be a wise move, and I couldn't have had a better start, nor been taught by a more able and kindly teacher. Prof's Chief Technician. William Cooper, was a short bespectacled man with a brusque and very direct manner. "So you're going out to work in the tropics with Dr. Heisch are you lad?" – he almost dared me to deny the charge. He went on – as if I hadn't spoken (I hadn't) – "and you come to work here – for no pay?" This was said in a tone of utter disbelief... "and you wish to learn parasitology techniques in only three months?" – his voice rose almost beyond audio frequency with these last three words.

He was a good actor, I'll give him that, but he couldn't sustain it for long. He suddenly smiled and said, "We should be able to teach you quite a bit in that time – but you'll have to work extra hard. Now lad, how much do you know?" No point in bluffing here, I said... "To be honest, virtually nothing at all; I'm starting very much on the ground floor".

At this he replied, "Good lad, I like honesty, that's good; you will learn – but you won't start on the ground floor, but right at the very bottom – in the basement, lad", he chuckled. "that's where we'll start you. Now, slip on this lab-coat and follow me". Grabbing the proffered white coat I sped after him as he swept down the corridor to the lift. In the basement of the London School of Hygiene & Tropical Medicine, beneath the pavements in the street above, were the insectaries. The rooms were hot and humid (automatically controlled) and had netted curtains at each door. Large gauzed cages on tables held the different mosquito colonies while the breeding rooms nearby had long concrete benches on which sat many large earthenware bowls of water, each with a big clump of grass and soil to provide the micro-organisms on which the young insect larvae fed. The later stage larvae were fed with daily sprinklings of Farex biscuit meal. The pre-emergent pupae were picked out with a small glass pipette and transferred to a small bowl of clean water which was then placed in the appropriate cage prior to emergence as adults.

Bill Cooper wasn't always the easiest of people to work with; he rightly set very high standards but was a kind and a consummate technician, as Professor Garnham later acknowledged in his obituary. Earlier at the DIBD in Nairobi Prof. Garnham and Prof. Shortt had worked out the initial exo-erythrocytic cycle of development of the malaria parasite in man, i.e. in his liver cells and, secondly, inside the red blood cells, where the parasites grew and multiplied again, finally rupturing the cell and releasing new broods of young parasites to infect other red cells – causing the periodic 48 hour fevers. The final proof of the preliminary liver cycle could be obtained only by using a human volunteer. Bill Cooper volunteered to be infected with the relatively benign *Plasmodium ovale* malaria and later had a liver biopsy under general anaesthetic, the piece removed being cut into very thin slices on a microtome and stained to reveal the developing parasites inside the (Küpfer) cells lining the liver sinusoids – thus confirming the theoretical belief. Under Bill Cooper's guidance I learned to handle dangerous organisms with safety and confidence. This stood me in good stead later and I will always be grateful for his help at the start of my 'promising career'.

CHAPTER 5

Outward Bound

Sea voyage to Kenya – join DIBD – meet the team

A little later, one cold afternoon at the King George V dock in London, I walked up the gangway on to the Warwick Castle, found my way eventually to my cabin, stowed my case and went back on deck to take a final farewell from my brother, his wife, their two small girls and a couple of close climbing friends, both of whom subsequently went to work and live permanently in Africa. The last warps were being slipped when a palpable and audible throbbing started deep down in the ship as the main engines came to life. The gap between the grey hull and dockside began to widen – the lone figures on the wharf began to recede – "Goodbye uncle Roy – come back soon!" I could just catch the voices of my nieces. How soon would that be I wondered? Off at last – with a slight sinking feeling in my middle as I speculated what the immediate future might hold for me. I waved my last goodbyes to the tiny figures still standing there until they finally faded from sight.

I stood on the aft deck feeling the wind-blown spray on my face and the trembling deck (or was it my legs?) and watching the disembodied lights on shore fading inexorably astern as we stood down Channel in the darkness. Cold, wet and with nothing more to see, I went below to meet my cabin-mate, Peter Hall – a young dark-haired lad going out to convalesce with relatives in Nairobi, following major surgery for tuberculosis.

Despite the excitement of being in the process of starting a new career in another country, perhaps because of it, I slept very well in the comfort of a cabin (in contrast to a crowded mess-deck) and in a proper bunk. This, being less responsive to the movements of the ship and despite its comparative opulence, didn't quite measure up to my hammock on the 'Andes'. The evening meal was sumptuous – five courses with a complimentary bottle of wine (for the first evening only) – in a huge and well-appointed dining saloon. The general atmosphere was friendly and relaxing; most of the passengers were those returning to East, Central or Southern Africa after home leave – all eager to return to the warm sun and blue skies after wintry Europe.

The route took us down Channel, round the isle of Ushant and across the Bay of Biscay before passing Cape St.Vincent and taking the first on the left into Gibraltar, which we reached whilst having breakfast. Later, ashore, we stretched our legs in the bright sunshine, enjoyed the window shopping and exploring the famous Rock. The next stop was Marseilles with its huge ramifying harbours. A few of us made the long laborious climb up the Notre Dame de la Garde, up the endless flights of stairs to the gilded figure of the Holy Virgin at the top and took in the magnificent view whilst we got our breath back. We soon lost it again when we used the public toilets at the bottom!

By this time the bridge players aboard had identified one another and virtually disappeared from view for the rest of the voyage. They could sometimes be seen (and heard) holding their innumerable inquests and post mortems in what would otherwise have been quiet corners of the lounge or library. After Genoa, with its colourful but steeply slanting streets, we cruised smoothly down the coast of Italy – with Stromboli casting a rich orange glow in the darkening sky. Such a voyage, on a well-appointed ship with a contented social atmosphere, was a mini-world in itself although, perhaps, a little divorced from reality. Before the advent of satellite communications to all intents and purposes passengers were virtually incommunicado and there were lots of interesting people to meet and talk with; especially to learn as much as possible about the new country that had been injudicious enough to invite me. There were many kinds of deck sports and other ways to pass the time. Some of the more extrovert South African youngsters indulged in vigorous games of 'Buk-buk' – a kind of elongated leap-frog where one side forms a ridge with their backs while the other takes it in turns to run and try to land as far up as possible without falling off. Several of the contestants intermittently received appropriate first-aid measures for bruises and wrenched shoulders. The fact that the ship's sick bay housed a very attractive young nursing sister may have had something to do with the number of superficial knocks needing attention!

Ocean cruises were noted for their shipboard romances, and this one was no exception. Unfortunately, in those relatively unenlightened times, such things were frowned upon by the authorities to the extent that the ship had a 'Master-at-Arms', one of whose duties it was to patrol the ship after dark and put a swift end to any incipient hankey-pankey. All deck chairs were stacked away and secured for the night. The library of course was very popular, as was the bar.

Also, for me, there was the added pleasurable knowledge that I was on half pay for the duration of the trip out. In many ways I think it a great pity that such a pleasant and restful mode of travel had to give way to the boredom and discomfort of inter-continental air travel.

Leaving the straits of Messina the ship now headed out into the heavier seas of the eastern Mediterranean. One minute the relentless deck-walkers would be climbing slowly uphill; the next, as the bow fell into the trough, they would be trying hard not to break into a gallop. Waiters with loaded trays walked at grotesque and changing angles, along corridors, with accustomed ease while newcomers proceeded with exaggerated caution, clutching the hand-rails. Those with weaker stomachs tended to disappear altogether. Mealtimes, too, had their amusing moments – 'fielding' errant plates and cutlery. The Suez canal came next, with the ship gliding through what appeared to be long stretches of sand at seven and a half knots – the maximum speed allowed. At night huge searchlights mounted on both sides of the flying bridge lit up the way ahead and, by next morning, we had reached Port Suez at the southern end of the canal – with the monument of its originator Ferdinand du Lessops. By now the outside temperatures were very much higher and the ventilators were going full blast. Mid-morning coffee, hot chocolate and Bovril had now given way to iced coffee and soft drinks and most evenings were spent on deck – with film-shows and dancing under the stars being very popular and well-attended.

As we lay at anchor just off Port Suez, the usual 'bum-boats' made their appearance. (Pl.3) Trading over the side of the ship was started usually by the throwing up of an unripe banana tied to a length of fibre rope from the floating market stall below. This brought up the handbag, snake-skin, beads, copper and brass ware and other items – all of which could be had for a suitably staggering sum – unless you haggled. The stratospheric starting prices seemed to suggest the offer of a major share-holding in a seemingly lucrative company – which no doubt it was. The old hands on board greeted these opening moves rather like a game of chess, the trader being quite undaunted by their derisive remarks and the almost insultingly low offers made – both of which were clearly expected. The more affluent traders had more sophisticated vessels, many sporting a tall mast with a lateen sail. Once manoeuvred alongside the mast provided a convenient ladder up which the enterprising trader shinned to the upper deck – for face-to-face bargaining. One leg entwining the mast ensured a reasonably secure perch and left both arms free to indulge a wide range of gestures and, where needed, to shake a fist at any approaching competitors. (Pl.4)

After a short stop at Port Sudan we moved on down the Red Sea in oppressive heat, even the breeze due to the ship's movement bringing little or no relief. By now the land was closing in noticeably on both sides before we finally 'turned the corner' and by late evening reached the free port of Aden. The shops were all brilliantly lit, well stocked with goodies and very quickly filled up with eager passengers, all jostling for bargains and haggling furiously over prices. The satisfied smiles on the faces of the shopkeepers gave the impression that, no matter how much they allowed themselves to be beaten down over prices, they would still make a handsome profit! Cameras, watches and transistor radios were on most people's lists and all seemed well satisfied with their purchases. The next day we rounded Cape Gardafui, the north-eastern tip of Somalia, before turning south for the last leg of the trip to Mombasa, Dar es Salaam, Zanzibar, Beira and the South African ports. The approach from the sea to the deep-water berths in Kilindini harbour at Mombasa is a delight to the eye. Luxuriant and gracefully curving coconut palms, gleaming white coral sands, colourful flamboyants, pink and white frangipanni flowers, blazing red poinsettias and the mango trees, even the occasional gaunt 'planted upside-down' baobab trees, all provided a fitting backdrop to the beautiful blue-green sea.

The first 'tourist' to set foot in Mombasa was Vasco da Gama in 1498. From the time when it was sacked by the Portugese, two years later, it was the scene of almost continuous strife. Despite its strength the massive and heavily armed Fort Jesus, overlooking the entrance to the Old Harbour, was finally stormed in 1698 and the few remaining defenders, reputedly eleven men and two women, were killed. The Old Harbour is only a few minutes walk from the fort, down Vasco da Gama street with its finely carved ornamental Arabian and Indian doorways and beautiful minarets, similar to those in Zanzibar The old harbour is now used only by native and small coastal craft; (Pl.5) these are principally dhows trading between East African ports and India, Madagascar and the Gulf States. The largest of these ocean-going dhows, of some 200-300 tons, come into the Old Harbour between December and April when the 'Kaskasi' (north-east monsoon wind) is blowing. These very picturesque vessels, still built and rigged as they were centuries ago, with high stems, often elaborately carved, enter harbour with flags flying and their crews dancing to the beating of drums, carrying cargoes of dates, Arab furniture, Persian carpets etc. The dhows in Mombasa Old Harbour are still one of the most remarkable sights in East Africa (*Year Book & Guide to East Africa*, 1982, Robert Hale Ltd., London). Those contemplating the praiseworthy notion of travelling on one of these romantic vessels should perhaps note that the 'usual offices' sometimes consist of a simple wooden box, with a hole in the floor, slung somewhat precariously over the stern. Those diffident about using it in rough weather may be encouraged by the novelty of having the Indian Ocean as a built-in bidet and reassured by knowing that, should the whole affair become detached 'à la moment critique', its all-wood construction would probably keep it afloat indefinitely!

I was met off the boat by a small, rotund man with dark curly hair, large glasses, a bustling manner and a huge grin. This was Mark Furlong – Dr. Heisch's 'man-in-Mombasa'. Since it was already late afternoon, Mark drove me to the main railway station nearby and saw me into my reserved two-berth compartment. The elegant silver trains, pulled by the massive Garratt articulated wood-burning locomotives painted in the attractive deep red colours of the East Africa Railways and Harbours, left Mombasa daily at 18.15 hrs for the 13-hour journey up to Nairobi – climbing from sea level to over 5400 ft in 350 miles. Soon after departure the smartly uniformed attendant came in with a bedding pack which he rolled out on the upper bunk to reveal spotless white sheets, a pillow and a warm blanket. Having first lowered the window fully I then proceeded to lower a cold celebratory 'Tusker' lager while I sat back to enjoy the passing scene. After leaving Mombasa Island the train crosses the Makuba Causeway and immediately plunges through groves of coconut palms, mangoes and banana plantations as it starts to climb the coastal escarpment. The air was pleasantly warm and humid and carried the fragrance of spices, wood-smoke and the many scents of tropical flowers and shrubs.

It was also full of fireflies, myriads of which winked brightly in the rapidly fading daylight. Still too excited to eat much I ordered a light snack, sipped another cold beer and sat watching the lights and village fires as we made our way slowly inland.

These Garratt engines are equipped with a substantial 'cowcatcher' on the front and a huge and powerful searchlight mounted in front of the funnel. This lit up the track ahead and gave the driver a chance to avoid collisions with any elephants, rhinos and buffaloes whose paths it happened to cross. 'Elephants have right of way' is an old and wise East African dictum, as those who have had the misfortune to run into them, usually at night and often near Voi (close to the Tsavo National Park), will know to their cost. Usually covered in dust (at that time from the dirt roads) elephants were particularly difficult to see in the car headlights at night.

To see better I incautiously leaned out of the window and was rewarded with a hot and stinging smut in the eye; this reminded me that Garratt engines are, or were then, wood- burning locomotives; but they are still magnificent beasts and admirably suited to the job of pulling long trains from the coast to the uplands of Africa.

Some years later, when working in Zambia near the Mosi-oa-tunya ('the smoke that thunders' – a far more imaginative name than Victoria Falls!) I came across the very sad sight of several old Garratt locomotives, complete with their huge tenders, at the 'railway-engine graveyard' in the sidings of the Livingstone Sawmills. They were standing forlornly among long lines of old rusting locos and delapidated coaches, all in various stages of decay and neglect. In his book 'The man who loves giants' the well-known artist David Shepherd, who has made so many fine paintings of elephants and other African wildlife, has also made some wonderful sketches of this railway 'graveyard'. He describes how he was given one of the old locos by President Kaunda and had it shipped back to England, to see out its days on the East-Somerset line – bringing great pleasure to many people besides himself.

Next morning, while breakfasting in the elegant dining car, with its huge observation windows, I feasted my eyes on the sight of Mount Kilimanjaro – a huge snow-covered plum pudding, some 80 miles away across the plains, showing up clearly in the limpid morning air. In the foreground and grazing unconcernedly, close to the track and seemingly oblivious of the passing train, were hundreds of zebras, wildebeests, hartebeests, giraffes, and the ubiquitous Thomson and Grant gazelles. A truly magnificent sight; and one, alas, probably now gone for ever.

Amid the press of people at Nairobi station and a rich mix of sounds, colours, smells and activities, I was hailed by a large bespectacled man with freckled face and cheerful grin. This was Arthur Harvey, the Chief Technician at the Division of Insect-borne Diseases, under whose aegis I would be working. The Medical Research Laboratory, with the DIBD on the upper floor, was within easy walking distance of my hotel (the 'Fairview') and I was immediately impressed with its pleasant semi-rural location opposite the big Jomo Kenyatta general hospital. During the morning coffee break Dr. Heisch introduced me to the other members of the unit. Dr. George Nelson (now Emeritus Professor of Parasitology at the Liverpool School of Tropical Medicine) had recently joined the DIBD after service as a District Medical Officer in Uganda. Elinor van Someren was a mosquito taxonomist of world renown who specialised in classifying/identifying the 'Culicine' mosquitoes (*Culex* and *Aedes* genera); she had acquired her expertise by drawing each species in detail and committing it to memory.

The African support staff had all been well trained and were magnificently led by Silas Achapa – the Senior Technician. Silas was always smiling, never upset or angry and always willing to help – his experience was vast and he was well liked by all. The DIBD was fortunate indeed to have such a highly talented and pleasant staff member.

The Senior Entomological Field Officer/Biologist (my immediate boss) was Bill Grainger, a pipe-smoking Irishman with a relaxed and pleasant demeanour and a quiet sense of fun; like all members of the DIBD he spoke fluent Kiswahili but his was particularly 'safi' (clean/pure) similar to that spoken in Zanzibar and along the coast. He spoke softly with a ready grin and was understandably well liked by all the staff, expatriate and local. Later I was allocated bench space in a large shady room which I shared with a huge bearded giant of a man – this was Charles Guggisberg (affectionately known by all as 'Guggi') a Swiss zoologist from Bern. Apart from his official activities as a mammalologist with the unit, Guggi spent most of his time photographing and writing about wild animals. Being something of an authority on the African wildlife he was much in demand for escorting parties round the National Parks (of which East Africa is rightly very proud) and giving lectures. A skilled photographer he marketed his many excellent colour pictures through a local studio in Nairobi.

Dr. Christopher Teesdale was the helminthologist, working mostly on the epidemiology of schistosomiasis (Bilharzia). This is one of the more debilitating worm diseases and is caught when the actively darting and wriggling larvae (cercariae) released into standing or sluggish water by certain snails, penetrate the skin and migrate to the deep mesenteric veins of the bowel (*S.mansoni*) or bladder (*S.haematobium*). The male and female worms lie (*in copula*) together in the portal veins of the liver. The eggs, migrating out through the tisses of the bowel or bladder, cause the typical bleeding associated with this disease. When away from the scientific scene Chris. Teesdale was a keen cricketer and played at a fairly high standard for the well-known 'Kongonis' team in Nairobi.

Below us, on the ground floor, was a biochemistry laboratory the staff of which were headed by another very remarkable and dynamic individual. Dr. Martin Case had gained double first-class honours degrees at Cambridge in biochemistry and physiology. After graduating he had joined a research team led by Professor Haldane. Martin had been one of the volunteers who had gone inside H.M. Thetis, a new submarine that had sunk off Liverpool, during preliminary sea trials, with the loss of more than 90 technicians and crew. The aim of these scientist volunteers was to assess the nature of their death by oxygen starvation; they were monitored carefully and finally brought out semi-conscious, proving to those who had lost loved ones, that their death had been painless and in sleep. Martin was also a gifted musician – a fine pianist and a noted oboeist with the Nairobi orchestra. From time to time the day would be enlivened by liquid scales and trills on the oboe, floating up from downstairs, as he warmed up for an evening concert. Dr. Geoffrey Timms, the eccentric Director of the Medical Research Laboratories, was notable for his broad smile, savage sense of humour, a very large straw hat and an unwavering insistence on driving everywhere in a very old, but still immaculate, Model T Ford... CLUNK! – the sudden metallic crash some 10 yards behind us made us both start, caused the car to rock dangerously and memory to make a two milliseconds jump back to the present. The door of the huge lion trap had obviously fallen but both Donald and I were sure that it must have been badly set and had fallen on its own. We had earlier considered that it was not particularly appropriate for the task and now hesitated before going over to reset it. But we had to be sure, so we pushed through the dense undergrowth and shone the torch at the trap. What greeted us was a deep-throated growl and the green eyes of a large and very angry leopard, one whose clear intent, were it free, being to disembowel us both before regaining the nocturnal sanctuary of the Langata forest. With the torch to guide us we walked back to break the news, the barking dogs waking the night-watchman who stumbled off to wake the household. The Leakey family came out to inspect the catch and we all sat around drinking coffee and chatting.

The next morning the Nairobi National Park staff came out with a lorry to collect their trap. First a large tarpaulin was tied over the cage, to quieten the still angry leopard, then it was loaded on and driven out to the Athi Plains, close to Lukenya along the Mombasa road. In these craggy outcrops leopards abound and are constantly swooping down to take dogs, sheep and goats from the farms at the bottom. The tarpaulin was removed, the tail-gate dropped down and a rope fixed to the top of the drop door. This was then passed over the bough of a nearby tree and led back into the cab. With a good strong pull the door rose a couple of feet and in a blurred yellow and black flash the leopard hit the ground running and was soon lost to sight amid the ground cover.

CHAPTER 6

Bush work

The DIBD – the District Commissioner dispenses justice in a local native court

Much lower down the academic scale, and with everything still to learn, mine was a relatively low-key existence. After a few weeks of familiarisation with the DIBD and under-studying Arthur Harvey, who was soon to go off on home leave, I was sent off 'on safari' to a place called Tseikuru as part of my initiation. At that time my only experience of the African bush had been our RAF navigation exercises in Zimbabwe and, vicariously, through the 'Tarzan' films, with Johnny Weissmüller (as Tarzan the Apeman) swinging effortlessly for vast distances on strategically placed lianas – sometimes with Cheetah, the chimp, sitting on his shoulder. One half expected him sometimes to lose his grip and to crash down out of sight to the forest floor, as most of us would have done! But, if he did, it was doubtless discarded on the cutting-room floor!

The road to Tseikuru went out of Nairobi first through the coffee-growing areas of Kahawa (Kiswahili = coffee) and Kiambu to Thika – the site of the famous Blue Posts Hotel and the picturesque Chania Falls. Elspeth Huxley's books 'The Flame Trees of Thika' and 'The Mottled Lizard' provide fascinating, amusing and poignantly evocative accounts of this part of Africa at the beginning of the last century; they also paint an impressive picture of the lives of the early settlers in Kenya and of their struggles to survive in the face of a variety of daily difficulties and, sometimes, dangers. At Thika we swung away eastwards, taking the road leading on to Garissa and, eventually, on down to the coast at Malindi. This road passes the controversial Yatta Furrow – a huge scheme to channel water from the Athi and Thika rivers into a flat arid plain, in an attempt to provide better agricultural conditions and opportunities for the Wakamba people. Shortly after the war the Wakamba had asked the Machakos District Commissioner, George Brown, to make extra land available to them for settlement. The land they wanted was occupied by many rhinos which had become a genuine menace, damaging the natives huts and crops and frightening anyone wandering about at night. J.A. Hunter, a Scottish white hunter, was given the job of clearing the rhino from the whole area – described fully in his book '*Hunter*' by Hunter.

On reaching a small town called Mwingi we left what had passed for a main road and turned north on to a smaller track which almost passed for a dried up-river bed. By this time the pleasures of travel on such roads in a short wheel-base Landrover were fast losing their appeal. Much of this journey was spent practising my fledgling Kiswahili with my two African companions, Ezekiel, an elderly, cheerful and perky character always grinning and Soloman – just the opposite, a quiet, shy man with an occasional gentle and seraphic smile. Both had been instructed by Dr. Heisch to use not one word of English to me during the trip. In its wisdom the British Colonial Government rightly insisted that all expatriate staff members acquire a good working knowledge of this mellifluous and very useful lingua franca, emphasising this intention by withholding all annual salary increments until the Standard Kiswahili examination had been passed and this achievement officially gazetted.

Tseikuru had been identified as an important focus of kala-azar (visceral leishmaniasis) a disease where the parasites in the blood are engulfed by the scavenging white blood cells (phagocytes) of the reticulo-endothelial system (spleen, liver, lymph nodes, bone marrow etc). The spleen gradually enlarges owing to the enormous increase in the R-E cells – many of them parasitized. Without proper treatment death may be quick or delayed – from a few weeks to about 2 years. There was growing concern at the rising number of cases and Donald had the difficult task of definitively identifying the vector – in this case a small hairy 'sandfly' (*Phlebotomus*) and, if possible, any wild animals that may be acting as a reservoir. Once in the infected area the sandflies were collected from as many different sites as possible, specifically identified (mainly by the shape of the filter at the back of the mouth, examined under the microscope) and dissected to look for the developing motile parasites in the front part of the gut. As with the mosquito vectors of malaria... "the female of the species is more deadly than the male"... since it is to nourish the developing eggs that the blood meal is needed – and during the collection of which the infection is passed on in the saliva. Although kala-azar is found in the hot arid regions the sandflies rest in such cool shady places as the insides of termite hills, in which they can be found in the upper parts of the tall ventilation shafts in the late evening. They are also found in rock holes and in river-bank holes made by birds. Using a small sucking tube the crevice or hole is probed with a thin stick and any sandflies can be seen in the torch beam with their short hopping flight and hairy wings.

The African staff were past masters at collecting these lively insects (Pl.7) – catching about 20 or more to my single specimen. The interviewer's words... "the Africans would have to teach you.." rang clearly in my memory as I quickly recognised their expertise. They were to teach me a very great deal, not all of it technical, during the many happy years that I was priveleged to spend working with them.

Some weeks later Donald and I had to return to Tseikuru (Pl.6) – this time to assess the disease situation in Usuene, a small satellite field station some 15 miles from Tseikuru on the bank of the Tana River. After another long and dusty drive we arrived at dusk, lit the pressure lamps, cooked dinner, enjoyed a couple of cold beers from the ice box, whilst sitting out under the stars, and later slept like logs. Whilst I was packing the Landrover to leave for Usuene (Donald was staying to organise work in and around Tseikuru) a runner arrived with a note from the local Chief, asking if I could give him a lift to Usuene, as his own Landrover was off the road with broken half-shaft. We crossed the dried-up river bed on the far side of Tseikuru and began the hour's drive, during which the Chief explained that he had only recently been appointed by the Government and was going to Usuene to meet the local Chiefs and village elders and afterwards to invite them to a celebration 'ngoma' (dance). There was a small Government rest-house built of lime-washed mud with a thatched roof and open sides giving magnificent views over the Tana River some 50 yards away and 50 feet below us.

The party started soon after dusk and went on for 2 days and nights. The dancing was raw and the energy expended impressive; most had adorned their legs, ankles and arms with bracelets of Fanta and Coca-Cola bottle tops threaded on to string loops. A few had whistles, others had drums of different sizes and pitch. The magnificent rhythms and cross rhythms from the drums were hypnotic and, when combined with the whistles and the murmuring 'shak-shak-shak' of the bottle-top bracelets, as they swayed back and forth stamping, blowing the whistles and, occasionally breaking into the vertical bouncing jumps typical of the Masai and Watutsi dancers, they were irresistible. I went down to watch but finished up joining them – the circle opening immediately to let me in. Two pressure lamps and a dozen or so hurricane lamps cast an eerie light over the sweating, leaping bodies and the clouds of dust raised by the stamping feet. When finally I stopped to nip back and rehydrate

I found that I had been dancing, almost non-stop, for over 2 hours. I slept well that night!

A day or so later, on our way back to Tseikuru, it was evident that there had been rain; there was that rich warm smell of freshly moistened sun-parched earth. As we came to the top of the slope leading down to the river by Tseikuru, it was clear that it had only recently flash-flooded; the river bed was a beautiful glistening blue-brown colour, still wet and reflecting the colour of the now clear sky. At the bottom of the slope I switched off and got out to check the state of the river-bed – on foot. But the Chief stopped me saying... "It's OK – we can cross, just follow that track there" pointing to a thin line of footprints leading diagonally across to the other side. 'He should know' I thought and slipping into 2nd gear and engaging low ratio started down the bank into the river bed... We were about half way across when the wheels began to lose traction and the Landrover sank slowly down into the mud – until the tops of the tyres disappeared from sight. 'Not many AA or RAC boxes in these parts' I thought – 'probably not even a serviceable tractor either'.

But I hadn't allowed for the Chief. "Wait" he said, opening the door and jumping down into the mud; then putting two fingers into his mouth he blew an ear-piercing whistle in the direction of what appeared to be a totally deserted Tseikuru village – some 200 yards away. As if by magic hundreds of villagers appeared and we were soon surrounded as by a swarm of ants. Inwardly cursing that I didn't have a cine-camera to record this extraordinary event, I watched dumbfounded as some thirty or forty villagers lifted the vehicle bodily up out of the mud and began pushing and dragging it to the other bank. I've since wondered what the AA or RAC man would have made of it and the catchword comes to mind… 'but I know a man who can'! The Chief just smiled and said "Thanks for the ride".

The next safari was another kala-azar investigation, this time in a focus centred on a place called Marigat on the Tigerri River just south of Lake Baringo in the Rift Valley. The DIBD had established a sizeable semi-permanent camp there in which staff could live and work for periods of up to a year or more. A large mobile laboratory was parked in the shade of a huge tree on the river bank and, with the fly screens up and all windows wide open it was a pleasant place to work – cool and free from the ubiquitous flies. It was equipped with gas, lighting, sinks, benches and even running water – provided that you filled up the roof tank periodically to make it run. We lived in tents while the more permanent mud huts were being built. These huts had a smooth cement floor and a grass thatched roof which attracted gheckoes and the smaller (thankfully) climbing snakes – which never harmed us and which we came almost to ignore. When properly adjusted to give a clean smokeless flame the kerosene fridge worked well despite the heat outside.

We found that the evaporation from a large wet towel draped over the top gave it a significant boost, as did the delightfully cold beer for us at the end of the day's work! The mosquito net was a necessary nuisance since it restricted the air-flow at night. But later, when the rains came, often very suddenly in the middle of the night, we would find ourselves moving the beds around to find the dry spots – where the water wasn't pouring in through gaps in the thatch. One could then throw a waterproof sheet over the net and go back to sleep – to sort it all out in the warmth of the early morning sunshine – much more sensible!

Whilst we were at Marigat Donald made a valiant attempt to breed sandflies, putting the eggs into small earthenware pots which were kept moist and in darkness – i.e. resembling the conditions inside the river-bank holes where sandflies were breeding and living naturally. He constructed a small electrical thermo-couple device to measure the atmospheric temperature and humidity in the natural breeding places and tried to replicate these inside the earthenware pots. This was almost successful but failed to complete the life cycle into adults. It was interesting and informative to watch his skill in dissection – showing the developing leishmania parasites in the anterior part of the insect gut. Having no previous entomological experience I was also intrigued by the method used by Donald to identify the different sandfly species. The head was cut off the dead insect and placed overnight in a solution of sodium hydroxide. This dissolved away all the soft parts leaving the harder filter at the back of the throat (the buccal armature) clear. This was then placed in a drop of fixative gum on a glass slide, rotated into the correct position and a thin glass cover-slip placed on top. When this hardened the sample could be viewed under the microscope and the details of the buccal armature (shape, number and arrangement of the 'teeth' etc) could be seen and used for specific identification.

One afternoon, while I was in the middle of an afternoon siesta, recovering from an all-night sandfly biting catch among the termite hills beside the road up to Kabernet, Paulo came to my tent to waken me and say "You have a visitor Bwana". I staggered to the tent door, wiping the sleep from my eyes, to be greeted by a burly, wide-awake and decidedly cheerful man, with bright eyes and disarming grin.

This was 'JB', Her Majesty's District Commissioner for this part of the British far flung empire, (as it then was) and living in a splendid and spacious house across the river at Marigat. "Sorry to wake you, young Rickman" he said, very successfully concealing his sorrow, "If you're not too busy tomorrow you may like to join me for a couple of hours. I'm trying a case of serious infidelity in a nearby village – and it will be a new experience for you." Although not entirely devoid of contact with the seamier side of life (having spent some months going round the back streets of Calcutta on brothel patrols whilst in service as a mechanic with the RAF police – when flying training ceased at the end of the war) – this was certainly something new. He went on: "If your Kiswahili is up to it – you may be able to follow the proceedings, since it will be conducted in the local lingo. Come over to my place about 10 am tomorrow – now back to sleep with you". With a last cheery grin and wave he climbed into his staff car, crossed the ford and vanished in a cloud of red murram dust.

In its wisdom H.M. Government had stipulated that all who came to work with the then colonial service in Africa (and presumably in other overseas territories) must pass the basic Standard Kiswahili examination, within two years of arrival, before gaining any regular annual salary increments. Although I had been studying this beautiful and expressive language for several months, as an essential prerequisite to becoming 'Tropical Diseases Consultant to H.M. Government', as I hoped, getting to grips with the seeming multiplicity of technical tasks had competed for my time and attention.

The following morning 'His Lordship's car, with its uniformed driver, came to collect me. Having shaved and put on clean shirt and shorts, even polished my shoes, I climbed aboard hoping that despite still being in 'scruff order' I wouldn't be too noticeable. I was greeted by the District Commissioner – "Glad you could make it, young Rickman; I think you might enjoy seeing a little dispensation of British justice by Her Majesty's humble and obedient (I had some doubts about both qualities!) representative". We drove up to the village to find some 100 or more men (mostly) sitting in a circle in the shade of a huge mango tree. Chiefs and Village Headmen and Elders were in padded chairs or wooden seats; lesser mortals were sitting either on long benches or on large wooden logs that had been dragged into place; those of still lesser consequence were sitting cross-legged on the ground. Fortunately the District Commissioner and I were invited to occupy two of the padded seats.

The central area had been carefully swept clean ready for the speakers – the custom being that only those who had gained possession of the special orator's wooden staff could speak. Those wishing to do so would raise an arm in request, which was usually long ignored – such is the joy derived from many a spoken word! By putting my nascent Kiswahili into overdrive and concentrating furiously I was able to get at least the gist of what was going on. The Senior Chief opened the proceedings with a formal welcome before plunging into a long and detailed discourse of the crime under study; this was an affair where a very young third or fourth wife of one of the Village Headmen had (understandably!) fallen for the attraction of a much younger and doubtless more virile villager. As they had been caught *in flagrante delicto* – such legal niceties as returning the sheep and goats paid as the bride price and the imposition of a penalty payment on the doubtless impecunious but still grinning miscreant were to be discussed. After a little while I looked across at the District Commissioner next to me and saw, to my horror, that he had slipped back in his seat, his legs were stretched out and his official solar topee was down over his eyes and covering his face. I was horrified to think that, at such an important occasion, he had fallen asleep! But no-one else seemed to have noticed and when all the worthies had voiced their opinions, denials, mitigating factors and criticisms – no doubt adding their supreme confidence that H.M. District Commissioner would support their particular opinions – he slowly pulled himself up, requested and was given the orator's staff and walked out slowly into the middle of the circular auditorium. Speaking (as expected) in beautiful and fluent Kiswahili, he quickly ran over the essential features of the case, each point being met with a general stamping of feet in approval. At the end he resorted to the art of mimicry – the African's delight – as I supposed imitating the behaviour of those closely involved. Immediately he had the whole assembly shaking their shoulders and roaring with laughter. When all was quiet again he gave his judgement which, it appeared, was fully endorsed by all and shown by more vigorous stamping of feet and nodding of heads. I had the impression that he had highlighted the obvious attraction that a handsome and virile young man would have for a young woman in servitude to an old man with three other wives to keep satisfied and an over fondness for maize beer.

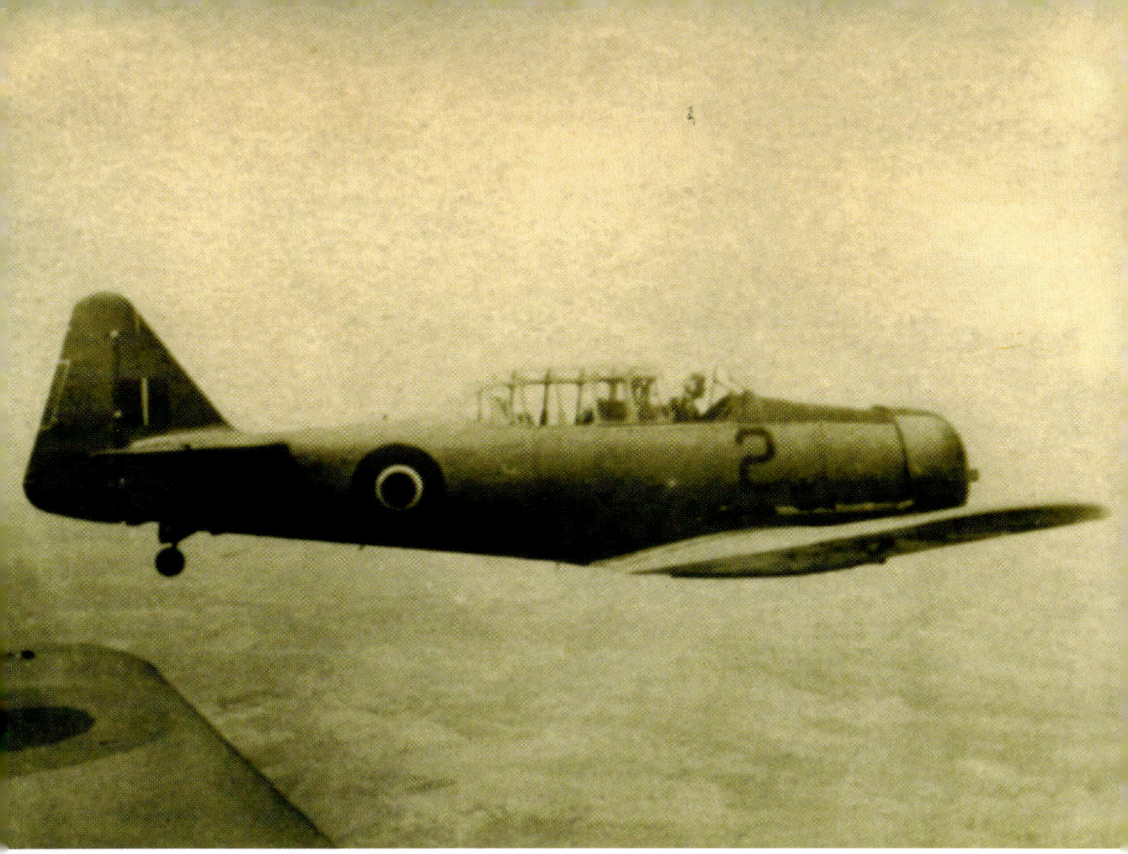

Above: *Plate 1*. Formation flying in 1945 - Roy flying solo in a Harvard IIa
Below: *Plate 2*. The Svellnos glacier in Norway (L to R: self, Len and Peter)

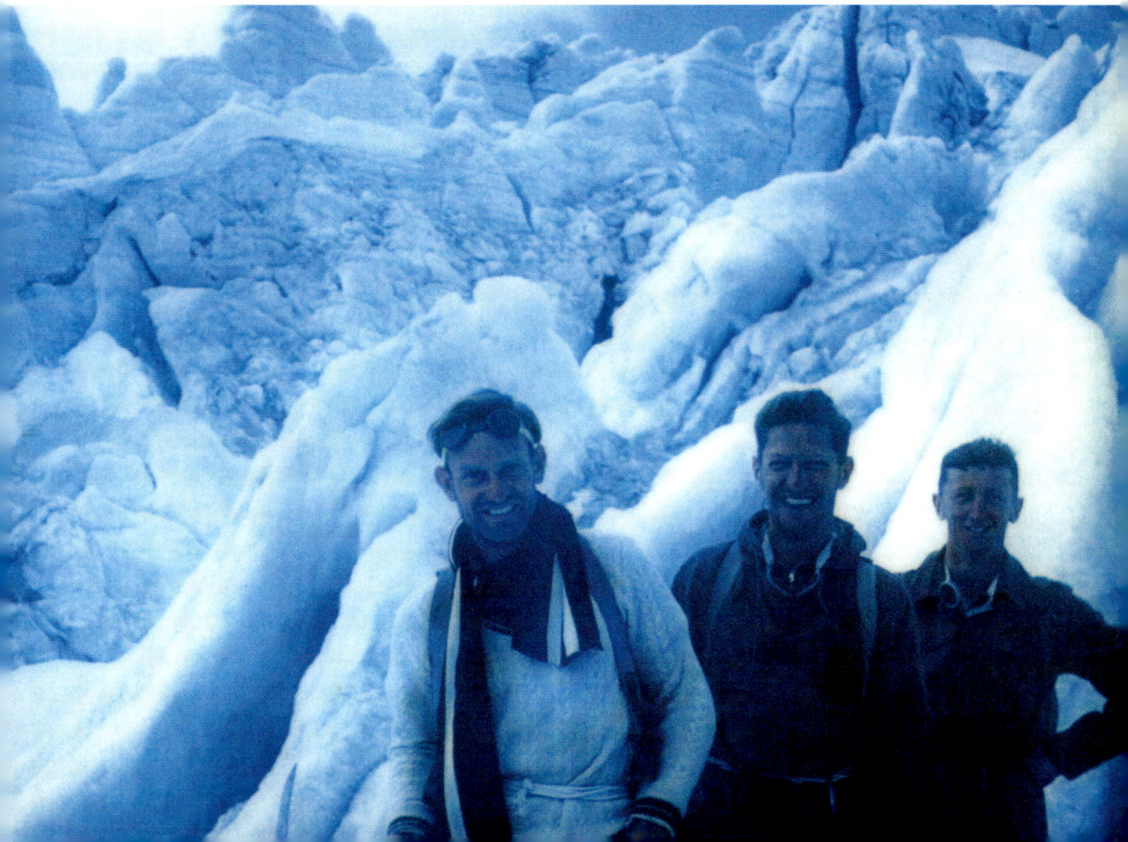

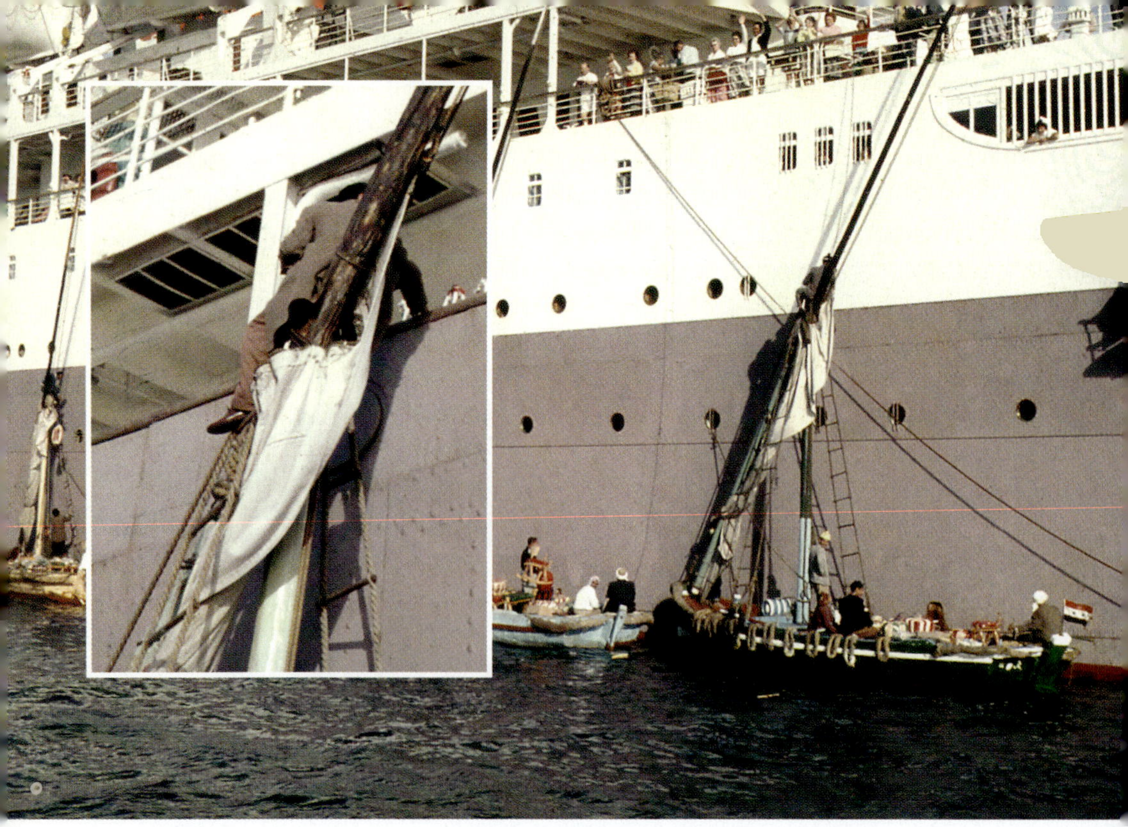

Above: *Plate 3.* Egyptian traders alongside *Warwick Castle*, Suez
Inset: *Plate 4.* Higher-level trading alongside the *Warwick Castle*, Suez
Below: *Plate 5.* Old harbour, Mombasa – with ocean dhows in from Persia

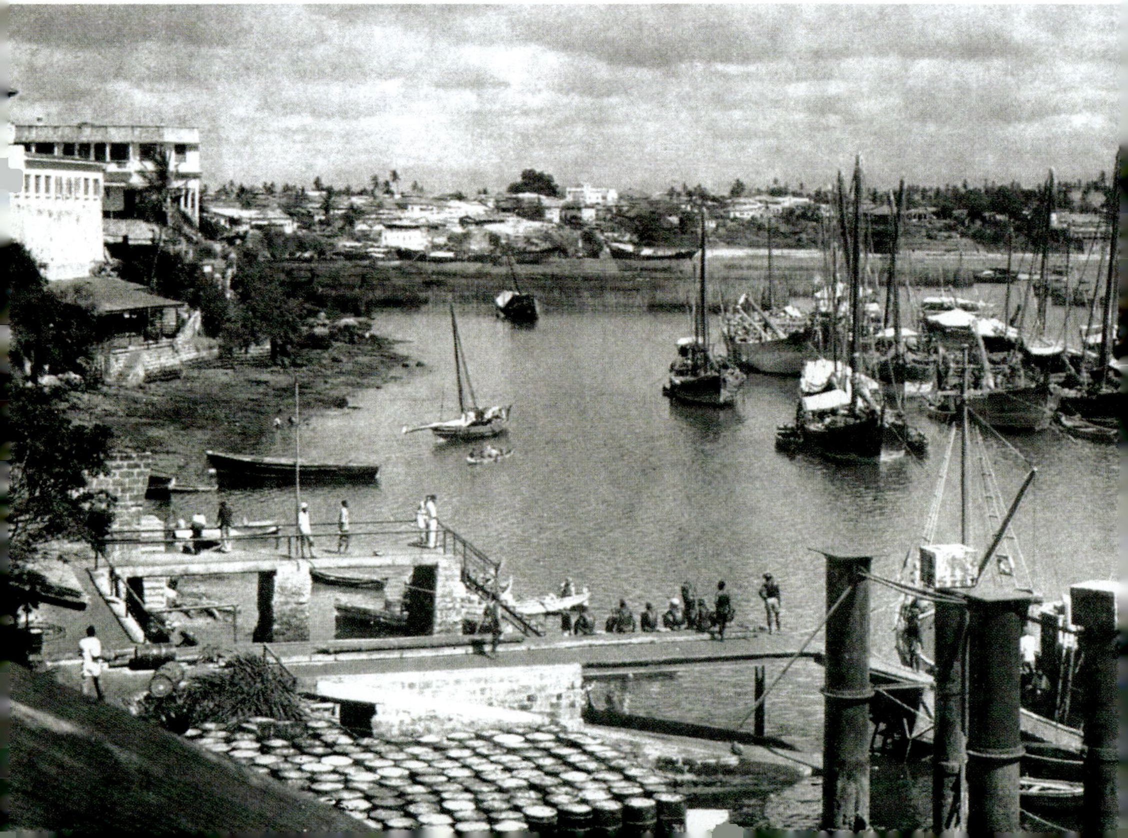

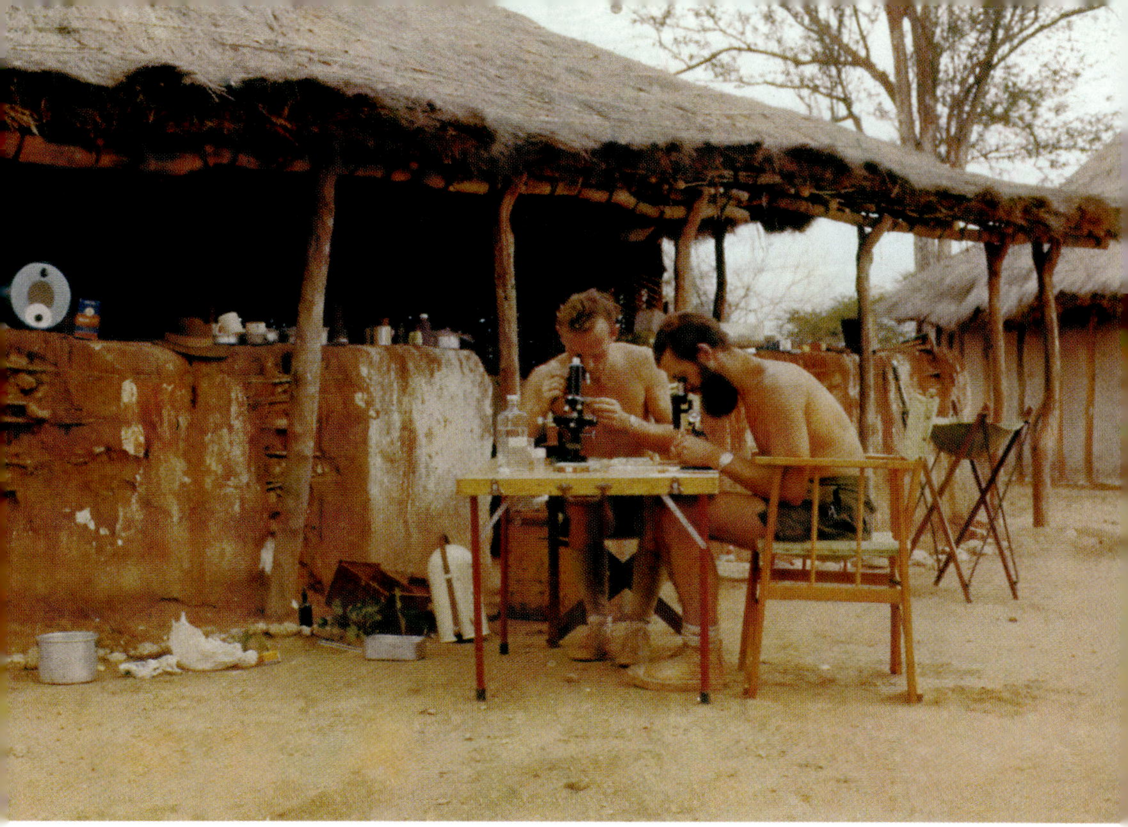

Above: *Plate 6.* With Donald Minter – microscopy at Tseikuru (note 'Saucepan' radio).
Below left: *Plate 7.* Catching sandflies in river-bank holes at Marigat, Kenya.
Below right: *Plate 8.* Lambwe Valley Field Survey Team en route

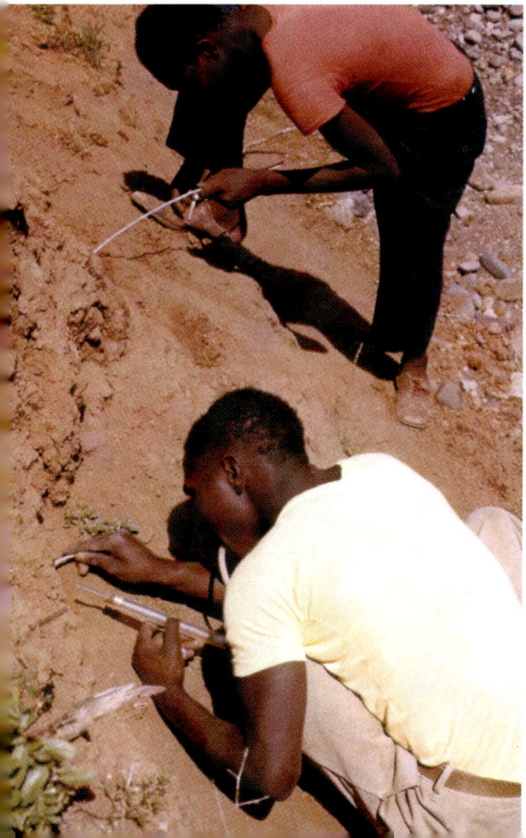

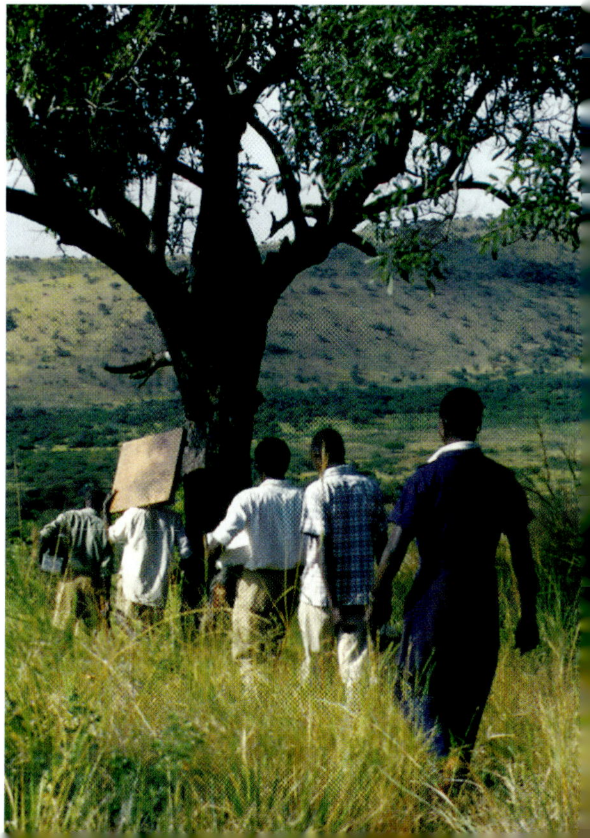

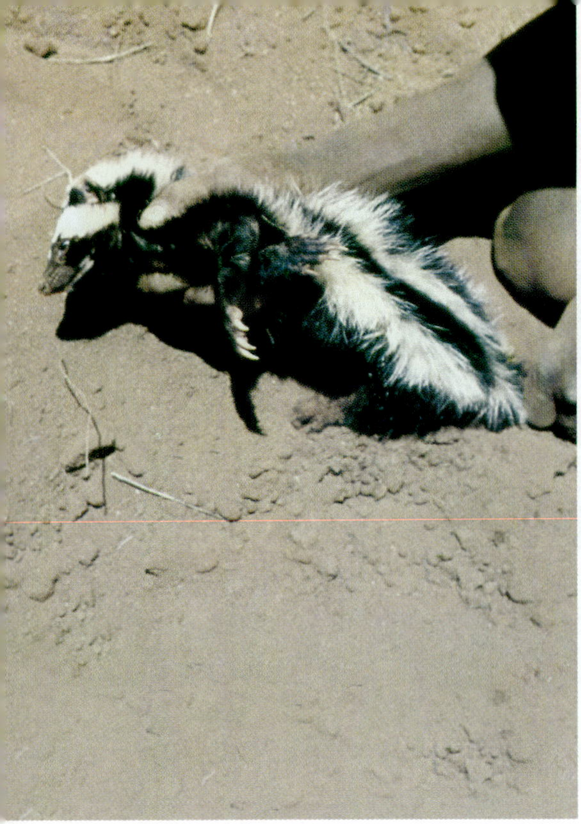

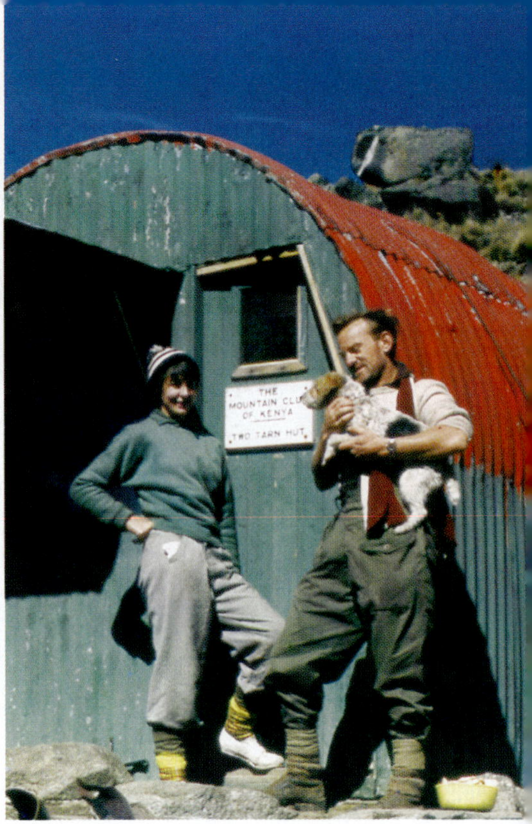

Above left: *Plate 9.* A 'zorilla' (African skunk) caught by Karissa Kikoi, DIBD, Kenya
Above right: *Plate 10.* Elspeth, Roy and canine at Two Hut Tarn, Mt Kenya (15,000ft)
Below: *Plate 11.* Setting box traps (L to R: self, Synema, Matata and Glayva

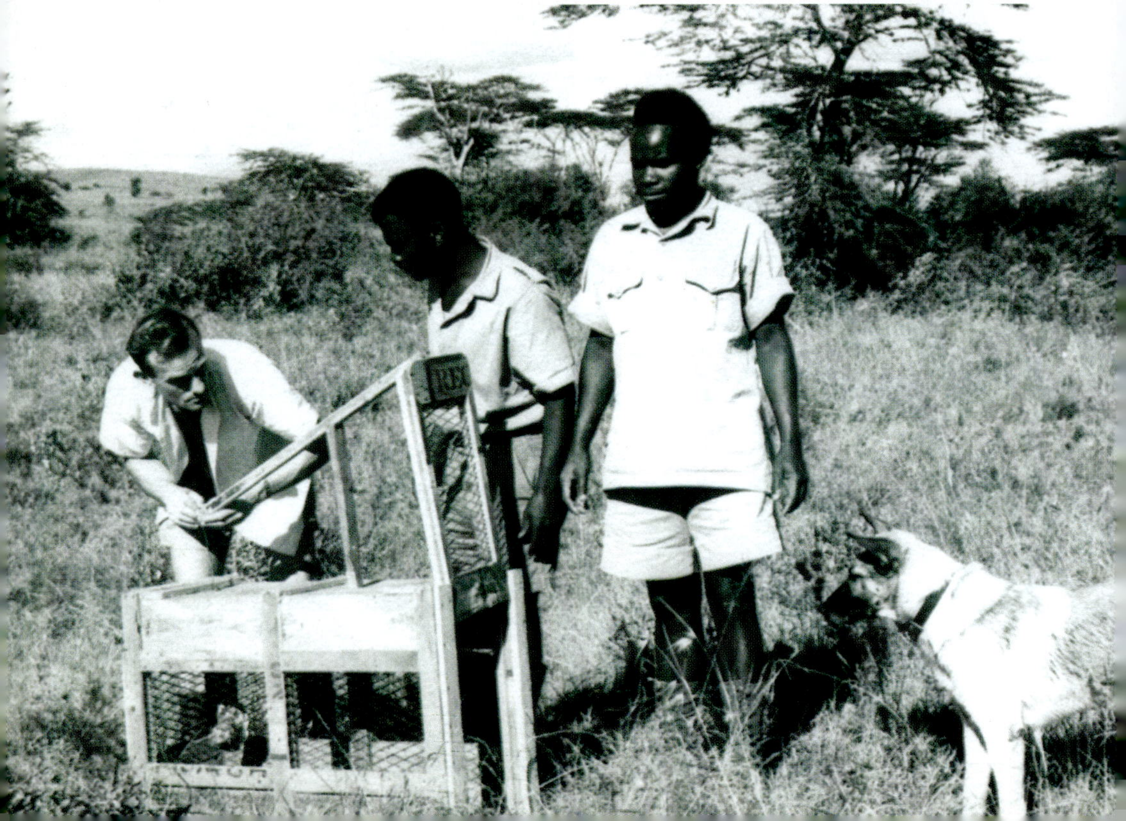

CHAPTER 7

Learning Curve

Field studies on Visceral leishmaniasis – animal trapping with biologist Bill Grainger and his team.

Soon Donald decided to extend the sandfly catching area to include Kampi ya Samaki (Fish camp) at the southern end of Lake Baringo. Here a young couple, David and Elizabeth Roberts (a retired crocodile hunter and a wonderful stand-in for Johnny Weissmüller's Tarzan) had developed a thriving fish catching and packing industry – sending the succulent lake-fish (Tilapia) packed in ice, down to the markets in Nakuru and Nairobi. Subsequently Tilapia found their way into the British supermarkets. Leishmaniasis cases were also coming from villages across the river, along the road leading up to Kabarnet – a cool 'Shangri–La' perched on the crest of the Kamasia Hills with fine views of the great Rift Valley on both sides. Kabernet had a few shops and a small hospital run by Dr. Brian Strangeways-Dixon a young English physician. The road from Marigat up to Kabernet was not made up or regularly graded and was something of an assault course – even in a Landrover. In several places, where the road crossed fast-flowing streams coming down from the hills, it was necessary to spend time remaking the road, putting some of the heavier boulders back into place so the vehicle could pass. Crossing the main drift at Marigat could be unpredictable and even dangerous at certain times of the year. This occurred when the heavy rains fell on the main catchment area around Timboroa, where the equator crosses the main Nairobi – Uganda road at over 9000 ft. The rapidly swelling river would slowly gather speed and by the time it reached Marigat, would come roaring through the narrow gorge, just upstream from the drift, as a frightening 4 ft tidal wave, running at about 12-15 knots. Carried along with this rushing brown torrent were many logs and small trees picked up en route. Any pedestrian, cyclist, or even a car caught on the drift at such a time, would be lucky to survive and it would be several hours before a crossing could safely be attempted.

We visited Kami ya Samaki fairly regularly, usually to buy fish or have a swim – despite the crocodiles which, although plentiful there, seemed not to attack man. David and Elizabeth and their children seemed to swim there every day without harm. Perhaps knowing that David had earlier been a keen crocodile hunter, they kept a healthy distance. In the centre of the lake is a large island much favoured by the local Njemp fishermen. They paddle across the lake in their home-made canoes which they build with strips of local balsa wood. These canoes are pointed at the bow, open at the stern and are only about 12-15 inches deep. The fishermen kneel inside and propel themselves by means of balsa wood scoops tied over the hands. Because balsa wood gradually becomes waterlogged they are almost sinking when they reach the island and have to leave the canoes to dry out in the hot sun before they can safely be used to the undertake the return journey. If not – it's a long swim!

Sadly only a few months after our arrival at Marigat, and whilst Donald and I were both working away in bush, David Roberts went down with a high fever and soon afterwards died, reportedly from a fulminating attack of cerebral malaria (*Plasmodium falciparum*). At that time, and before drug-resistant malaria strains became a widespread medical problem, such infections were easily curable, if diagnosed and treated early. It seemed a terrible shame that such a physically strong young man should die in such a way. Several years later I returned briefly to Kampi ya Samaki to find Elizabeth still running the camp which had been enlarged as a tourist attraction. A fine house had been built on the water's edge and the beautiful gardens filled with oleanders, hibiscus, frangipanni and cascades of multi-coloured bougainvilleae. The favourites with the children were a huge turtle and a very full-grown cheetah which, like a tame dog, was patiently cooperative, playful but completely safe.

Donald having identified a likely 'candidate vector' sandfly species (*Phlebotomus martini*) it was necessary to study its behaviour in more detail by monitoring its frequency and determining its peaks of man-biting activity. This was studied during a continuous 48-hour cycle, in several different locations, by recording the number of bites per hour and the species involved. At first we felt (and must have looked) 'right charlies' – sitting around termite hills with sleeves and trousers rolled up high, with torches and sucking tubes at the ready, waiting for them to arrive. Whilst away on one of these 'biting cycle' studies, the river at Marigat flash-flooded just before the manager of Rowland Ward (the 'trophy specialists' in Nairobi) arrived with his wife and two children to visit the District Commissioner, whose house was at Marigat on the other side of the river. By this time it was dark, they were all tired and, with the river in full spate, a crossing was out of the question. Fortunately Paulo, who was my acting house steward, remembered that I had earlier pinned a 'Welcome' card to the flap of my large tent with full instructions as to where the visitor would find food, drinks, beds and bedding. Paulo took this card out to the visitors and guided them back to comparative comfort – with a pressure lamp, a full fridge with food,milk and plenty of beers and soft drinks and mossie nets. When I returned a couple of days later they had stuffed my fridge with many 'goodies' plus a full bottle of malt whisky and a letter of thanks. This sense of freedom to leave 'front doors' open, with a standing invite to the passing stranger, was quite normal in East Africa at that time and one of the many compensations of life in bush. Nothing was ever stolen during our absences – which speaks for itself!

Some time later, after another of these all night sessions, I was awakened just after midday by Paulo, who told me that a group of Njemp warriors had arrived with a badly wounded man – and could I please help? When I went out to investigate the Njemps were sitting in the shade of the tree by the mobile laboratory – drinking cold water which Paulo had thoughtfully provided. Gradually the story emerged. They had been out hunting since dawn, looking for antelopes or other animals to kill for food. They had chanced upon a solitary lion which they encircled and, Masai-like (to which tribe they are closely related), they started to attack it with their spears. Finally, thinking it almost dead, one of their number had gone in for the 'kill'. But he was in for a very unpleasant surprise; the roles were now reversed. The lion, far from being moribund, sprang on him, burying both sets of claws just below the shoulder blades, and had ripped up two large flaps of flesh from his back.

His companions moved in quickly and killed the lion then tried to do what they could for their wounded comrade. Although deep in shock and doubtless in considerable pain, he hadn't bled profusely. They wrapped him tightly in the blanket he was wearing, made a crude stretcher from saplings and started to carry him back to Marigat. Since the movement of the stretcher rubbing on his lacerated back was more than he could tolerate he decided to walk the 10-12 miles back to our camp – in the heat of the day, supported by his friends and still wrapped in the dirty blanket After such an achievement he deserved to survive! I re-bandaged him as gently as I could, replacing the blanket with a clean white bed sheet and had them lift him carefully into the Landrover. We sat him on a mattress and packed him round with pillows and cushions and allocated two of his friends to look after him during the journey. I drove as fast as

I dared up to the hospital at Kabarnet and handed him over to Brian who, unfortunately, had only just finished one operation and now had to go straight into another. The injuries were quite extensive and required much cleaning and disinfecting as well as stitching and dressing. This was successfully completed some hours later and he was put to bed. It was several days before Brian brought him down again in his Landrover to Marigat. By this time the victim was all smiles and thanks and one couldn't but be amazed at the physical strength, courage and endurance of these nomadic tribesmen who, like their famous Masai brothers, are highly respected by those who know them and the simple spartan life they lead as wandering herdsmen tending their cattle.

Rodents were strongly suspected as being reservoirs of kala-azar and this finally proved to be the case in East Africa. The decision to examine ground squirrels (*Euxerus* species) meant a move further north to the Kerio Valley; this was on the other side of the Kamasia Hills beyond Kabarnet, in the western part of the Rift Valley. Bill Grainger with his animal catching team had already set up camp in the Kerio and I was asked to take a 30 cwt Bedford truck with supplies and to stay and work with Bill and his team to widen my experience.

Taking turns at the wheel, the DIBD driver and I left Marigat, drove up to Kabarnet then down the other side, crossing the bridge over the impressive Cheblock Gorge. Dusk fell as we followed the dirt road that crosses the valley and climbs up the Elgeyo-Marakwet Escarpment to Tambach and eventually across the Uasin Gishu to Eldoret. We looked carefully in the headlight beams trying not to miss the small track that would take us north from this main road for about 20 miles up the Kerio Valley to where Bill Grainger was reported to be camped. About half way across we saw a solitary figure standing there by the road-side, a tired and trusty Soloman. He had been dropped there earlier to make sure that we didn't miss the turning – a tacit reflection of Bill Grainger's opinion of my navigational skills!

With Soloman to guide us we continued up the track and after some 15 miles, could see a single bright light ahead. As we drew nearer we could see that it was a pressure lamp strung up outside a large tent and illuminating a very relaxed Bill Grainger sitting with his faithful pipe, a glass of amber fluid in one hand and book in the other. He got up and walked over to greet us – but not before he had spoken to Soloman in Swahili, "Thank you, Soloman – I told the cook to save you some chakula (food)". Then, turning to us, he said with a slow smile (which more than 40 years on for me still characterises this quiet and gentle man)… “So you finally managed to track us down then – welcome! It’s good to see you. Did you have any problems on the way?” “None. other than night blindness” I replied. “Thanks for sending Soloman to help us – otherwise we would probably have ended up in Tambach”. He offered me a chair and pushed across a goodly measure of neat whisky and a flask of cold water. “This will ease some of the travel stiffness and help you sleep after you’ve had a good wash down. When did you last eat – you must be hungry?”.

We shared a light but magnificent meal that, at that time, couldn’t have been bettered – a fillet steak from a waterbuck, shot earlier that day to provide food for the team, one that the chef at the Ritz would have been proud of! We sat and listened to the BBC news on his little battery-powered EverReady ‘saucepan’ radio. A single length of wire with a stone tied to one end had been thrown up over a high branch to provide an excellent aerial and the batteries seemed to last for ages since the set was used only mornings and evenings for the news bulletins. “I’ve put you over there” said Bill, pointing with his pipe stem to a large open flysheet pitched nearby. “You won’t need a tent – it’s too warm – but use your net there are plenty of mossies about – sleep well”. The mosquito net was soon rigged up and I slid quickly under the single sheet and was soon asleep. It had been a long and tiring day.

Ten minutes later, or so it seemed (actually it was a couple of hours before dawn) – I was instantly awake, tense and with all my back hairs standing on end. It was bright moonlight; what had woken me was the full-blooded roar of a lion, very close by, then another and another – equally close. I must confess that, by this time, I was lying there petrified, with ears straining to hear the first sounds of the beasts approaching through the bush. There was nothing between me and them but a flimsy mosquito net. I still cannot remember how long this lasted but, eventually, a combination of physical and mental exhaustion must have won the day for I fell asleep again and woke to the noises of a busy camp preparing to breakfast in beautiful morning sunshine. Washed and dressed I walked across to join Bill who was sitting with his first cup of tea. “Ready for some tea young Rickman?” he said with an impish grin as he pulled out another chair for me. “How did you sleep? I hope the lions didn’t worry you too much”. I confessed that I thought I had heard something but was too tired to get up and see what it was. He grinned again, not believing a word of it, and said, “My fault – I should have warned you that they were about. But there’s no danger, they don’t come into the camp. But remember, they roar only after they have eaten

– not before!”. Again I was lucky in my mentor; I learned much from Bill – as I am sure Dr. Heisch intended me to do.

For the next few weeks I worked with him and his team of animal catchers – fitting in where I could. For the smaller rodents Ngumbao and Synema, the ‘old hands’, would first select some long stems of grass and weave these into long tapering cones each about 3 inches in diameter at the entrance. Once the rat ‘runs’ in the grass had been spotted they were followed up and, invariably, led to the main nest. This was often in an old termite mound in the middle of a large bush. The cones were then laid in the runs, with the pointed nose nearest the nest, and were then covered with grass to make them virtually invisible. The trappers then spread out in a wide circle and, at a given shout or whistle, would start stamping and beating the ground with sticks as they walked towards the nest. Any rats in the undergrowth would race along the nearest run and dive headlong into the cones – the harder they pushed to get free the tighter they were held. Small samples of blood were taken – usually from the tip of the tail – after which they were wiped with disinfectant and released back into the bush. Other larger rodents like the ground squirrels were caught in small wire cages baited with peanuts or by digging down into their burrows.

On one such occasion one of Bill’s animal handlers, Karissa Kikoi, was digging down one entrance when he turned his head aside quickly in disgust as he pushed up sand to block the hole. Having taken a deep breath he continued digging to reveal a black and white striped ‘zorilla’ or African skunk (Pl.9). He held it out at arms length with head averted, whilst a small blood sample was taken after which it was released. The smell from its defence glands was most unpleasant and extremely powerful. Many of the termite hills were inhabited by colonies of mongooses which could often be seen playing about on the top of the mound in the evening sunshine. But these termitaries are also home to many snakes so it paid to be very careful when working in or near them and remembering always never to put ones arm inside.

The work with the ground squirrels was duly rewarded when a strain of kala-azar was isolated from them and successfully cultured in a blood-agar medium. This was later used by Dr. Clinton Manson-Bahr to make a vaccine which, in turn, was successfully tested soon after. Another active focus of kala-azar was at Loboi, at the top end of what was then Lake Hannington (named after Bishop Hannington, of the Church Missionary Society, who in the early part of the last century, was killed by local tribesmen while travelling in that area). It is now called Lake Bogoria and is noted for its hot springs (maji moto = hot water). On our first drive there with the 30 cwt truck we drove too close to the lake and became stuck in loose sand. Nothing daunted we stripped to the waist and set about digging ourselves out, lying on our stomachs and using hands and arms to pull the sand from in front of the sump. With the truck once again back on terra firma, and since we were now covered in sand and sweat, we stripped off completely and ran into the lake to freshen up. The many flamingoes there could have warned us (if they hadn't been laughing their socks off) that it was a soda lake. We emerged looking like 'fairy queens' covered in glistening crystals. We rubbed off what we could and hurried back to camp in record time for a good strip wash in the cool water of the river at Marigat.

One evening soon after our arrival at Marigat, Donald and I were sitting out enjoying the cool night breeze and watching the stars, before turning in, when we were both shocked to hear a blood-curdling scream coming from the gorge just above the drift. It sounded like a coloratura soprano being done to death in a terribly gruesome fashion. It was only the mating call of a tree hyrax (*Dendrohyrax arboreus*) the listed enemies of which were eagles, leopards, genet cats and which now include startled medical researchers! (I joke – for they are truly delightful creatures!).

CHAPTER 8

Tapeworms - Trapping and Two-Tarn Hut

The Rift Valley – a pointless leopard killing – Mt. Kenya – and the eccentric Raymond Hook

It wasn't long before I was recalled to Nairobi to work with George Nelson on a new project – tapeworms! These are common parasites of man in many parts of the world and, in Africa, the 'beef tapeworm' (*Taenia saginata*) is particularly prevalent in areas of livestock husbandry. The very high rate of infection of cattle in some areas with the cystic stage (*Cysticerca bovis*), is a cause for great concern because of the down-grading, sometimes even the total condemnation at slaughter, of the 'measly' carcase meat for human consumption. Previous efforts to eliminate the parasite, by treating the people and improving health standards, had not been very successful. Many of the cattle owners were convinced that the cysts seen in game animals were identical with those found in cattle, and that wild animals must be heavily involved in the infection cycle.

Medical H.Qs had been approached by a number of local farmers complaining that, because of the down-grading of their cattle at slaughter, they were losing vast sums of money. It could be expected that wild antelopes and other animals of the open plains could be carrying human-infective cysts – especially in areas like the Masai plains where cattle shared the grazing grounds with large numbers of wildebeest, giraffe, Thomson and Grant gazelles, kongoni (hartebeest), eland and zebra. Because of the shortage of water and green grazing, most of the farms in the Rift Valley were more suitable for ranching then for dairying and many of them were located close to Masai grazing areas.

On examination some of the farm staff were found to be infected with the beef tapeworms and it was almost certain that the gravid worm segments, full of eggs, were being picked up by the grazing cattle from the faecally contaminated grass around the cattle-holding 'kraals'. In the absence of public toilets within running distance, the nearest patch of (non-prickly!) grass usually serves the purpose – the hot sun and the industrious scarab (dung) beetles do the rest. My own preference when 'communing with nature' was a small spade and a toilet roll, stamping the earth back in the temporary cavity to avoid attracting flies. But if staying in the area for some time it pays to remember which parts of the bush have already been visited!

The farmers were all convinced that the game animals which shared their land for much of the time were the real culprits and were bringing in fresh infections to their cattle. Two main areas were selected for this study – 'Kenplains' a mixed dairy/ranch of some 22,000 acres on the Athi Plains opposite Lukenya, some 20 miles from Nairobi down the Mombasa road. The other was 'Akira Ranch' – a huge 95,000 acre cattle-ranch in the Rift Valley midway between the Masai town of Narok (on the Loita Plain) and Naivasha. Akira took in the extinct volcano of Ol Ongonot (Mt. Longonot) and the 'Hell's Gate' area adjoining Lake Naivasha. We were also asked to sample some of the many spotted hyaenas (*Crocuta crocuta*) at the Ngong township on the south-western edge of Nairobi. Ngong faces out on to that part of the Rift Valley that stretches southwards to embrace the soda lakes of Magadi and Natron and continues down to Lake Manyara and the breathtakingly beautiful extinct volcanic caldera (explosion crater) of Ngorongoro in Tanzania – which is now a famous tourist spot because of its abundance of wildlife coming in from the even more famous Serengeti plains.

We started the study at Kenplains, pitching our tents just outside the hedge which surrounding the large single-storey home of the owners – Mr. and Mrs Graham. We examined all of the farm staff and treated those few that had tapeworm eggs in their stools. This was followed by a visit to the local Kenya Meat Commission's abattoir and meat processing factory at Athi River to collect recorded infection rates of the Kenplains cattle. It was also important to learn the correct meat inspection techniques from Dr. Ginsberg, the Senior Veterinary Scientist at the abattoir, since we would later be examining some of the wild animals on location. For routine inspections two cuts were made, one across the masseter muscle of the lower jaw: the other across the gluteus maximus of the upper thigh. Any cysts present showed up as pale yellow or white pea-sized lumps and these would be squeezed out, pressed between two glass slides and examined under the microscope. The invaginated embryo tapeworm egg with its hookless suckers identified the beef tapeworm cyst with certainty.

For the wild animal examinations, the Game Department had loaned me a double-barrelled Greener 12-bore shotgun with plenty of SG and SSG cartridges. There was also a .22 rifle with long, high-powered Alfamax cartridges – for use on the smaller animals. Bill Grainger had sent two of his animal trappers to work with me, Synema and a younger lad named Matata. He had the build of an Olympic athlete and a fair turn of speed – as we were to witness a little later.

Like many of the wives of Kenya farmers at that time Mrs. Graham kept a wild animal orphanage for young, abandoned and sick animals, which the farm staff found out on the plains and brought in for her to look after. These were kept enclosed for safety but had the free run of the garden for most of the day. One of the more delightful occupants was a bottle-reared baby giraffe which, like all young things, was affectionate and playful but often had difficulty in deciding how best to manage its ungainly legs. The Grahams also kept open house to other wild animals, which could come and go as they pleased. One Saturday evening, when my assistants had gone back to their families for the weekend, I was enjoying an early evening cold beer with my hosts, in their spacious sitting room, when the curtains were suddenly pushed out and two fully grown serval cats (*Felis serval*) came in through the window and jumped down into the room. They circled the room a couple of times then made for a large empty sofa and curled up there side by side.

"Don't touch them" said Mr. Graham, quite unnecessarily, "Just ignore them". This was a mite difficult to do since their purring made normal conversation almost impossible; I wondered what the form was if one of them were to decide that a strange lap might be worth exploring! The servals are long-legged, fast-running cats of the African savannah and can weigh up to 20 kg; nocturnally active for the most part, they are beautiful beasts with a yellowish brown coat with black spots, a short black banded tail and a dark brown bar across the back of the large upstanding ears. Immediately Mrs Graham emerged from the kitchen wearing heavy leather gauntlets and carrying some pieces of raw fresh fish; they both ran to her rearing up on their hind legs and reaching for the fish with their paws. Once fed they gave a high-pitched plaintive cry then sprang up to the open window and disappeared back into the night.

One morning, as we were about to start trapping and examining the carnivores, Mr. Graham arrived at our tent to say that one of his horses, that had been sick for some time, had died the previous evening. He suggested that if he left it out on the plains, away from the house, I could sit out by it and shoot one or two of the hyaenas and jackals that the carcase would soon attract. My Landrover had been fitted with a powerful spotlight on the roof controlled from within the cab. This meant that I could drive around the ranch at night, with Synema or Matata sweeping with the light, on both sides of the tracks, to find the few animals, both herbivores and carnivores, that we needed to examine for the survey. They were both expert at identifying the different species caught in the spotlight – mainly by the eyes and the type of movement of the animal. The dead horse was loaded on to a farm truck and carried a mile or so from the house out on to the open plains and later, when it was dark, we drove out to the spot to see what, if anything, was happening.

Having arrived there I switched on the spotlight and immediately picked up a dark shape beside the body of the horse, about 30 yards away. It turned towards us showing two large bright green eyes and the typically sloping back of a large spotted hyaena, which had been biting into one of the back legs. Synema held the light steady while I slipped out of the driving seat, loaded the shotgun with SSG cartridges took quick aim and fired. When I looked again the hyaena was flat on its side and quite motionless, having been killed instantly. Impressive evidence of the power of its jaws was the sight of one of the horse's thigh bones – bitten clean through.

The herbivorous animals examined at Kenplains included Thomson and Grant gazelles, impala. oribi and steinbok; the carnivores included leopards, hyaenas, jackals, genet cats and one or two species of vultures. In the antelopes we found a few cysts but none that was human-infective. With the carnivores we dissected out the intestines which were pinned out under water in a large dish filled with black wax and dissected carefully, looking for the Taenia tapeworms and (even more carefully!) for the very much smaller and infinitely more dangerous hydatid disease worms (*Echinococcus granulosus*) which are found in dogs, wolves, jackals, foxes and other carnivorous animals. Man is infected when he swallows eggs from the third (gravid terminal) segment; this is mostly in children who allow infected dogs, (which frequently lick themselves) to lick them around the face. The eggs migrate through the body commonly to the liver and lungs and other organs where they produce huge slow-growing fluid-filled cysts which can be difficult and dangerous to remove.

The hyaenas and vultures in particular were loaded with worms which came spilling out as a slowly writhing mass in the dissecting trays. (Please tell the cook – no tagliatelle today thank you!). However, since this was all valuable academic research material, it was preserved in labelled bottles of formalin and sent back to the laboratory – for others to evaluate. So far we had found no evidence of game involvement in the human tapeworm cycle; but we had so far looked at only the few animals that we had shot. Now we were about to start trapping some of the smaller carnivores. These included genet cats, mongooses (including the large swamp mongoose), serval cats, wild cats which were all caught in rectangular wooden box traps. These had double chicken wire sides and had a drop door held up with a thin stick balanced over a vertical sick in the centre (Pl.11). To this was attached a vertical wire which passed through a small hole in the top and ended in a hook. This was baited with a small piece of meat or leftover sausage – although this latter was rarely available!

We started by siting the boxes up among the rocks on the Lukenya ridge, opposite Kenplains. Climbers from the Mountain Club of Kenya climbed here every weekend – often accompanied by the Governor, His Excellency Sir Evelyn Baring or 'H.E.' as he was affectionately known. Standing all of 6 ft 6 inches he was a first class rock climber and climbed mainly with the club's top performers on the more severe rock pitches. Although a keen member of the Climbing Club myself, I was in a much lower class of capability but enjoyed climbing on the lovely sun-warmed rocks of lesser difficulty. This was typical leopard country and the lady (Miss Major) who owned the farm at the foot of the end bluff, known as Edinburgh Castle, had lost many dogs, sheep and goats to them. Her lounge was draped with several skins from predatory leopards which she had shot while protecting her animals.

Synema came into his own now – he was the expert at setting and siting the box traps, as well as handling the captured animals afterwards. Since most of these small carnivores were nocturnally active we set the traps at dusk and, to prevent any trapped animals from suffering exposure to the sun during the day, we checked and cleared all traps at dawn the next day, leaving all trap-doors closed until the early evening. One morning early, as we climbed the path to where we knew a trap to be, we saw that the door was down and excitedly began to speculate among ourselves as to what we had caught. However, as we came closer to it we found it empty. At first this was surprising but not when we noticed that the double chicken wire on the drop door had a large hole in the centre. On examining this more closely we could see small fragments of skin and some blood stains on the wire and realised that a fairly powerful animal had managed to break out. A couple of days later, in the same area, we caught a small female leopard in one of the larger box traps borrowed from the National Park. We soon saw that she had skinned part of the front of her snout and forehead – the culprit! When we approached the trap she had managed to lift the door up about 12 inches with her teeth but clearly couldn't escape. We covered her with a tarpaulin to shield her from the sun and loaded the whole thing on to the Landrover and drove out to the National Park, where one of the Senior Wardens later released her by attaching a rope to the trap door and looping this over a strong tree branch where, from the safety of the cab, this was pulled and the leopard bounded out and scrambled up into the rocks to freedom.

It is just possible that this young animal was the one that had frightened the life out of Synema only a few days earlier at Lukenya. On that particular evening, as we started to return to camp after setting the traps, Synema, at the back of the Landrover shouted that one of them had already fallen and banged on the cab roof shouting... "Ngoja kidogo, bwana" (hang on a minute, skipper)... "Milango ya mtego moja umeanguka (the door of one of the traps has fallen)... "nitarudi upesi kuutengeneza" (I'll slip back quickly and fix it). He jumped down and started back up the slope, weaving his way between the rocky outcrops and bushes. He reappeared 5 minutes or so later but was no longer his usual cheerful self and, even more strange, his flies were undone! When we gently drew attention to his gaping fly he grinned sheepishly and explained what had happened. He had re-set the fallen trap-door and turned to come back down when he decided to 'spend a penny' in a convenient bush. As he stood there singing quietly to himself., expressing his thoughts in the typical African sing-song recitative. he suddenly became aware of a pair of yellow-green eyes of a leopard looking back at him from within the bush. He said he didn't stop the sing-song, but changed the words slightly... "Hello, Mr. Leopard – how are you? Be at ease my friend, don't be afraid of me (that must have made it smile!) – I'm not going to hurt you – I'm just on my way home now – stay where you are – don't bother to come with me, I know the way – goodnight!". He backed slowly away until he thought it safe to turn then moved steadily down the track to the Landrover at the bottom – without looking back. In the distraction of the moment he forgot to do up his flies – perfectly understandable. Only an obsessive sartorialist would have acted otherwise!

Another engaging vignette of this philosophising African recitative occurred a few days later when I was sitting outside my tent at Kenplains, enjoying the cool of the evening and the slow swing of the southern constellations millions of miles above me. Before turning in I heard a faint continuously intoned sing-song chatter interspersed with whistles, tongue clicking and occasional grunting, gradually getting louder. Eventually an old, creaking ox-cart came trundling by, a small hurricane lamp swinging underneath lighting up two placid oxen. Sitting on the cart, with one leg dangling down between the shafts and keeping up this constant stream of encouragement to the two plodding animals, was the huddled form of the driver. Whether what he was saying was complimentary or mildly abusive mattered not, for they went on their way apparently unheeding; though I suspect that he was well aware that they might have felt strangely uneasy and vulnerable had he suddenly fallen silent.

To complete this phase of the work we next spent a few nights on the plains just outside the abattoir at Ngong township on the south-western outskirts of Nairobi. The meat inspector there had been recording abnormally high numbers of condemned cattle carcases, coming in from the surrounding farms, all heavily infected with tapeworm cysts. The local people told us of the trouble they were having with packs of hyaenas coming in off the plains, attracted by the smell of the carcases stacked up ready for incineration. George Nelson was keen to examine them also for evidence of the hydatid cyst tapeworms (*Echinococcus granulosus*) and Dr. Clinton Manson-Bahr, a medical specialist from the big Jomo Kenyatta hospital, offered his services as an additional marksman.

With Synema and Matata to help we tied one or two of the condemned carcases to the back of the Landrover and towed them round the plains for about 15 minutes then piled them together in a heap. We then withdrew about 30 yards, switched off all lights and sat quietly. George and Clinton were standing in the back, one on either side of the spotlight and resting their weapons on the cab roof. Clinton had a beautiful bolt-action Mauser .256 rifle acquired during the campaign in Ethiopia. George had the 12-bore loaded with SSG cartridges. The name 'laughing hyaena' wasn't new to me, but the sound when it came certainly was. The rippling gurgles and chuckles interspersed with grunts, yelps, screams and excited whimpers, coming out of the darkness, announced the arrival of the main guests at the feast. "Ready when you are", Clinton's whispered words were accompanied by quiet taps on the cab roof. All lights were switched on to reveal several pairs of green eyes looking up at us from the carcases. George and Clinton managed to shoot five in all before the rest ran off into the darkness.

A day or so later we set a large wooden lion trap loaned from the National Park down on the slopes below the Ngong township. This was baited with some of the condemned carcase meat and left overnight. Next morning as we approached the trap we could see that it was already surrounded by onlookers all curious to see what it had caught. It was yet another of the hyaenas, but during the night this one had chewed away most of the wooden parts of the trap and almost freed itself. Since we already had enough material we took it out into the plains, away from the township, where on release it gave a derisive 'whoo – oop' and loped away to safety.

No *T.saginata* tapeworms were found in any of the wild carnivores and only one herbivore, a wildebeest, was a found to have the typically non-hooked cysts in its muscles. This proved fairly conclusively that wild animals were playing no significant role in this disease. But before leaving Kenplains, to work at the Akira Ranch in the Rift Valley, we had one small study to complete – that of the Cape or Jumping Hare (*Lepus capensis*), many hundreds of which thronged the Athi plains at night. These beautiful little animals are like miniature kangaroos with a long bushy black-tipped tail, large ears, very short front legs and huge eyes which gleam like green saucers in the spotlight. They are entirely nocturnal and live in large underground burrows. They were reported to be infected with small round-worms transmitted to them by the fleas they carry in their coat. The method of catching them sounded simple enough – make a lot of noise to confuse them, then chase them on foot – with a torch in one hand leaving the other free to catch them by the ears. I tried this myself early on and was running flat out with the others when I put a foot into an ant-bear hole and went sprawling. I lay there in the darkness, thoroughly winded and without the torch, until the stars stopped gyrating. I found the torch and rejoined the others none-the-worse for the tumble and with 'Dr. Suntan's words still ringing in my head. "At the moment they will have to teach you". Touché!

By contrast, the athletic Matata had given chase to a highly mobile and jinking grey form, which he finally grabbed by the ears. He brought it over to the Landrover headlights only to find that it was an ordinary hare that he had run down! The catchphrase "I can't – but I know a man who can' again seemed appropriate Ant-bear holes were a common feature of these game plains and were certainly traps for the unwary. They could do great damage to the springs and shock-absorbers of vehicles, not to mention the luckless passengers.

One evening soon after, whilst doing the routine night circuit with the spotlight, we spotted a large pig-like animal with a long snout and very large ears. Alarmed by our noisy arrival, and even as we watched, it quickly dug itself down into the ground and disappeared out of harm's way – within a matter of 20 or 30 seconds. This was the aard-vark or ant-bear (*Orycteropus afer*), another strictly nocturnal animal, feeding mainly on ants and termites which they dig out with their powerful spade-like claws. They excavate and live in these large burrows which have many exits – all of them perfect Landrover traps. Although weighing up to 80 kg the ant-bear has many enemies;

these include the spotted hyaenas, many of which live in old antbear holes and which they must often share with rusting parts of Landrover front-end suspensions!.

Our next venue was Akira Ranch – a 95,000-acre cattle ranch on the Loita Plains about ten miles east of the Masai town of Narok. The ranch was managed by a huge Danish farmer and his wife, Tommy and Jytte Thomsen, and their four children. The assistant manager was another young Danish man – Jorgen Lange. They lived in a large rambling farmhouse surrounded by an acre or two of garden protected, against the many types of wild animals there, by a thick thorn hedge. To the west was Masai land,where itinerant herds of cattle were constantly moving from one grazing area to another. Since the Masai believe that Engai (God) made them custodians over all cattle, the presence of Akira's 5,000 head of prime beef animals must have been irresistible, especially when compared with their own less impressive and often less healthy beasts. Often the only thing to disturb the peace and serenity of this lovely part of Kenya was the soft rustling of the Akira cattle!

Tommy had his work cut out to keep the intruders at bay. One morning, after a particularly successful cattle raid, he drove out on to the plains to the major manyatta (camp) where he saw some of his cattle surrounded by a ring of admiring Masai. In his fury he snatched up their spears, dumped them in the back of his Landrover and drove off to see the local Masai Chief. Through an interpreter he told him that those responsible for taking the animals could have their spears back only when they returned the cattle to Akira. If they didn't he would personally shoot every Masai that he saw on his ranch. Knowing virtually no fear themselves they clearly recognised a kindred spirit and returned his cattle the next day. To help guard the cattle in their kraals overnight, Tommy had issued his cattle men with rifles, but despite giving them only blank cartridges, for their own safety as much as for the Masai, many and lurid were the tales and claims of how many intruders they had bagged!

But with the clear cloudless skies, once the sun goes down, the temperature falls rapidly and to keep themselves warm, and partly also to deter any predatory lions, the cattle-minders lit quite large fires inside the kraals. From time to time wind-blown sparks would catch the tinder-dry grass which, fanned by night breeze, could quickly spread. These extensive grass fires were a particular hazard and every effort was taken to minimize the spread once the fire had taken hold. We were called out several times to beat at the flames with branches. Bush fires are very common in Africa. Many are lit by the pastoralists just before the rains are due in order to get the benefit of the new young growth. Others are lit by hunters who set nets downwind before using the advancing fire to drive the animals into them. Some fires are truly horrendous and very frightening. Once flying back to Africa from Europe at night huge tongues of flame could be seen clearly from the plane flying at some 35,000 ft.

The work at Akira Ranch was extremely interesting, with a wide range of wildlife to sample – much of it at night using the spotlight and box traps. 'Hell's Gate' was a favourite spot though, being a narrow gorge between sheer cliffs for much of its length, there was little enough room to manoeuvre if charged by a buffalo or rhino – and there were plenty of both there at the time. Hell's Gate is now a National Park, and deservedly so. At the far end are fumaroles and, at the western escarpment cliffs, a regular witch's cauldron with sulphurous boiling mud constantly bubbling up. Circling above in lazy effortless flight on their eight-foot wingspan wings and nesting on the top of the cliffs, were bearded Lammergeier vultures. Many evenings were spent going round this huge ranch, sweeping either side with the spotlight; this gave us the chance to see some of the rarer purely nocturnal animals such as the lovely little bat-eared foxes (*Otocyon megalotis*) playing around their home in an ant-bear hole, the small, striped insect-eating aardwolf (*Proteles cristatus*) with a similar home – thanks to their aardvaark estate agent! Another fine sight was a herd of some twenty to thirty Cape elands (*Taurotragus oryx*) with their straight spiral horns and dewlaps swinging as they trotted along. It is said that, given the right circumstances, all antelopes are good jumpers – and this holds true for the eland, the largest of the antelopes. I had first-hand experience of this once when, driving slowly round a sharp bend in the famous Amboseli National Park, with the magnificent Mt. Kilimanjaro massif as a scenic backdrop, I surprised a solitary bull eland grazing quietly beside a large bush which I judged to be about 6 ft high. Caught thus unawares, it lifted its head, gathered itself and, taking only one or two steps, sailed over the bush – clearing it comfortably!.

These night circuits of the ranch with the spotlight became quite an attraction and the Thomsens had many visitors wanting to accompany us with these nocturnal 'game viewing' trips. These included some of the Scandinavian Airlines aircrews who, stopping over in Nairobi for their mandatory rest period, chose to spend it at Akira. Since their flightpath back to Europe passed over this part of the Great Rift Valley, soon after climbing away from Nairobi Airport at about 10 p.m. they would switch all the landing lights on and off in farewell salute as they flew over us off to the north. One evening, while sweeping with the spotlight, I picked up a solitary ostrich sitting motionless some 2 or 3 yards from the edge of the track. Instead of running at our approach, as I had expected, it sat perfectly still looking straight at us. We soon discovered the reason, first one little inquisitive head popped out from beneath her 'skirt', then another, and another, until she was ringed by some 20 or so baby ostriches – the twenty or so pairs of twinkling eyes forming a perfect 'bush chandelier' – a rare moment indeed! All that remained was to douse the light and move on – taking only the precious memory with us!

One weekend whilst I was away in Nairobi Tommy and Jytte's son Finn came out to visit them from his architecture studies in Denmark. To celebrate, Tommy decided to take him out for a night drive with the additional aim of 'bagging' a leopard if possible. As they passed one particular clump of bushes the spotlight showed up a pair of bright eyes and, moving closer, they could see it was a leopard. Tommy shot at it with his 9mm rifle and, although wounded, the animal retreated further into bush where they couldn't reach it. Tommy decided to follow it up – going round one side of the bush clump and Finn, his son, armed only with a .22 rifle, the other. Within seconds the leopard broke cover leaping on to Finn and knocking him to the ground. Rushing to the scene Tommy could only stand there helpless, unable to fire for fear of hitting his son as he and the leopard rolled around on the ground. With equal suddenness the leopard sprang off and once again disappeared into the bushes. Fin was rushed immediately to hospital in Nairobi and immediately admitted – he had been badly mauled. Now more than ever determined to kill this animal Tommy went out again in the Landrover the following night, alone, to the same spot and heard growls coming from deep in the bush when he shone the light. Resting his rifle on the open door he was preparing to fire when the leopard came straight at him. This time he didn't miss and the animal fell dead a couple of yards in front of him. Examining the leopard back at the house the reason why Finn escaped being killed, or at least disembowelled, became clear. Tommy's first shot the night before had severely damaged both its back legs. The fact that, even after lying all night in pain and stiffening up, it was still able to spring to the attack is testimony to the ferocity and power of these fine animals. Other than an ego-boosting trip such hunting would seem to have little justification; in this case it could so easily have cost him the life of his eldest son. As it was the 95 stitches that were needed to patch him up, to me indicated the cost, but not the value, of such a senseless exercise, one that Finn was lucky to survive.

It was whilst at Akira that I received a letter from my friend Dick

Brandram-Jones, the Agricultural Research Officer at Marigat, asking if I would like to join him and Elspeth, his fiance, climbing on Mt. Kenya. I had some experience of mountaineering in winter, both in Scotland and Norway, and when in Nairobi spent many weekends rock-climbing at Lukenya. I willingly agreed to join them although I thought it most unlikely that we would get anywhere near the summit, having no crampons, ropes, ice-axes or proper high altitude windproof clothing. The twin peaks of Mt. Kenya (Nelion and Batian), are first-class rock and ice climbs with heights of over 17,000 ft. – not to be undertaken by the inexperienced or ill equipped! Earlier, whilst week-end climbing at Lukenya I had chatted with a couple of climbers, of the Mountain Club of Kenya, who were practising abseiling (roping down) techniques in preparation for an attempt on the Mt. Kenya summit. The older of them was an experienced Austrian who had climbed much in the Alps: his partner, although younger and very fit, had done virtually no climbing at all. Accompanied by their two lady-friends they set up camp at the bottom of the main summit mass and next morning, before dawn, set off to tackle the summit (Batian), hoping to rejoin the ladies before dark. Delayed by the state of the ice on the little Diamond Glacier between the two peaks, they were late in getting back and daylight faded completely as they reached the final steep pitch separating them from the camp at the bottom.

They had only two choices – to sit it out through a long bitterly cold night, and complete the descent in the morning, or to tackle this final 500 ft pitch in the dark. They decided to press on down. The older man was half-way down the first abseil when the anchor rock, from which the rope was suspended, came away from the mountain and he fell to his death on the rocks below. The younger man also fell but, although landing safely on a small ledge, broke his leg in doing so. One of the ladies heroically raced down to the valley in the dark to raise the alarm, which must have been a terrifying experience in itself. Although the mountain rescue team reached the injured climber in record time, he died soon after from shock and exposure. Such a tragedy almost inevitably calls to mind some thoughts on this written by Geoffrey Winthrop Young, the doyen of early British mountaineers… "Mountain climbing is an adventure in which there is always an element of risk, even of danger to life. A man who climbs alone with a novice, a younger person or pupil, handicaps himself to an extent that should forbid him to attempt any but absolutely elementary climbing". This seems sadly relevant.

Mt. Kenya, a snow-clad mountain 17,085 ft and visible from Nairobi is a great peak seamed with some fifteen glaciers. It is geologically an old and deeply dissected volcano in a very advanced state of decay; the actual crater has disappeared. The remaining volcanic plug is of much-weathered nepheline syenite, some parts of which are ice fractured and clearly unstable. The mountain itself is clothed with magnificent forests of elder, camphor and yellow-wood; it also has bamboo at altitudes of 5,500 – 11,000 ft The circular tour of the mountain, from Nairobi and back is the most picturesque route in the Highlands of Kenya and covers some 360 miles. On the east side of the mountain at an altitude of 15,000 ft, and only ten miles from the equator, is a small lake surrounded by snow slopes where a sheet of ice 100 yards across exists all the year round.

But experience shows that the 17,000 ft summit of Mt. Kenya is not a place for beginners, although the rest of the massif offers wonderful views and recreation. Before starting the long climb up the valley we first spent a very interesting two or three days at Raymond Hook's farm at Nanyuki, at the foot of the western side of the mountain. Raymond was an interesting and eccentric 'character', his one eye, small goatee Africaner-type beard and a moustache stained yellow with snuff-taking gave him a real piratical appearance. He lived simply, with his sister, in a small but cosy farmhouse. His great knowledge of the mountain and its abundant wildlife had been put to good use in a number of different ways. Most notably he had crossed Arab stallions with zebra mares and his grounds were dotted with partially striped offspring. Raymond had been an animal trapper and collector and had a small zoo on his farm. He used to catch cheetahs, to indulge the whims of rich Indian rajahs, and he showed us some delightful cuttings from British newspapers supporting his claim to have taken cheetahs to London to race at the White City Stadium. The press photographs showed the cheetahs in full flight jumping over the backs of the streaking greyhounds. He was a good raconteur and gave me much valuable information about the rodents living on the mountain – which George Nelson had asked me to trap and bring to Nairobi. Raymond's brother, Commander Logan Hook, owned and ran the Equator Inn in Nanyuki which had a white line drawn through the bar coincident with the equator, so that in theory you could, if you were so inclined, stand with a foot on either side and have a drink in both hemispheres. Whether geographical purists would accept such an accurate demarcation of a line of latitude, however commercially convenient, is debatable. As we cartographical surveyors were given to saying... "one has to draw a line somewhere". Being an ex-submariner 'Mine host' clearly knew where it should be!

Raymond supplied us with a donkey to carry Elspeth up the long, wearisome and seemingly endless track up to the foot of the peaks and we were soon joined by a small party of climbers from Zimbabwe. At first the path led up through thick forest which abounded with wildlife and several times we heard large animals, probably buffaloes, crashing away through the undergrowth. Once there was a very strong smell of 'cat' at the foot of a heavily clawed tree. Bravely resisting the temptation to look up and find the cause we moved on, for a while at a markedly higher 'strike-rate' and with markedly larger paces. Once clear of the winding track we came out on to steeply rising open moorland, appropriately named the 'vertical bog' and covered with large elephant footprints filled with dark brown peaty water. We pitched camp in the dark, I pitched my small Black's 'Tinker' tent in one and, although initially cold and wet, slept well.

The upper slopes were dotted with giant groundsels and lobelias and eventually the snow-capped peaks and glaciers came into sight. Such is the scale of the mountain that we were all well-nigh exhausted when we finally reached the 'Two-Tarn' mountain hut (Pl.10) wanting only to drink and sleep. By this time I was almost totally lethargic and running quite a high fever, Feeling no better next morning, and in a futile effort to shake myself out of this lethargy and wake myself up, I went outside, stripped off and threw myself into the small shallow tarn, close to the hut. The sheet of ice was only a millemetre or two thick and so did no external physical harm – the temperature shock when I broke through into the water was something else. Fortunately I had enough strength left to nip back smartly into the hut, wrap myself quickly in a thick blanket, make some hot coffee on the primus and dive into the sleeping bag to recover before my violent shivering woke the others.

After a couple of days we made a slow descent using the compass in thick cloud and slithering over the huge tussocks of grass when we accidentally strayed from the path for a short time. We finally reached Nanyuki again in warm sunshine, pleased to be down but sad that we hadn't been fit enough to go higher. A far more interesting account of daring and initiative in climbing this mountain the book 'No Picnic on Mount Kenya' is recommended. It is written by two Italian prisoners of war who broke out of their P.O.W. camp near Nanyuki solely for this purpose – using home-made crampons, ice-axes and rope etc. It is a credit both to their ingenuity and their courage; it makes excellent reading and is a classic of its kind.

CHAPTER 9

Tick-Typhus & Travels

Infected with unknown wild virus – hospitalised – a beautiful nurse – Ian Bompas – visit Uganda and the Outward Bound school at Loitokitok, Mt. Kilimanjaro and Dar es Salaam

Soon after our return to Nairobi the DIBD scientists and staff had been asked to work on tick typhus – at the request of Medical H.Qs. There had been a worrying increase in the number of cases and many queries had been raised as to which were the main risk areas and how the infection could best be avoided. The hard (*Ixodid*) ticks that carry the infection were everywhere plentiful and an epidemiological study was decided upon. First, though, it was necessary to learn how to identify the different species collected from a number of different hosts. These included, horses, cattle, sheep, goats, cats and dogs, birds and also from the wild animals and birds shot on the Kenplains ranch at Athi River. Ticks were also collected from domestic dogs in and around Nairobi; most people being only to pleased to have someone de-tick their pets – free of charge!

The typhus organisms (*Rickettsiae*) are of a size midway between bacteria and the much smaller viruses and when put on to a microslide and processed with Machiavello stain they show up as tiny pink rods against the pale green or blue background. As part of the study Bill Grainger and his team of animal catchers visited several of the working areas, mainly to collect rats and other smaller mammals – an activity for which they had been specially trained for earlier studies on rat-transmitted plague in the old foci at Rongai and on the plains at the foot of Mt. Kilimanjaro. With Arthur Harvey now on leave in England it fell to me to carry out the routine sub-culturing of the typhus organisms originally isolated (obtained) from rat blood samples. Dr. Heisch had warned us that this is the dangerous phase and, because of the real risk of accidental air-borne droplet infection with the highly infectious 'Q' fever, we were all told to wear masks and gowns and to seal all windows and doors when making the isolations. Unbeknown to us, and confident that one or other of us would become infected, Dr. Heisch has thoughtfully reserved a bed in the local Infectious Diseases Hospital (IDH) – just in case.

One evening, a couple of weeks later, I started to shiver uncontrollably and found I had a temperature of 104°. After a quick phone-call, I was whisked away to the IDH, put to bed, given a large flask of squash and a couple of antipyretic pills. First thing next morning Dr. Lawes, the Director, came in grinning, armed with a syringe and bottle – to take a large volume of blood to send to South Africa for specialist analysis. I shared a room with Ib, a young Danish boy, and we were well looked after. The food was excellent, the fever slowly subsided and there were plenty of interesting staff and patients to talk with. But although the IDH seemed fully occupied at the time, there was much worse to come. Soon afterwards there was a sudden and increasing inrush of patients as a result of a polio epidemic and the IDH was soon filled to overflowing. Extra beds were made up on the verandahs and these and other spaces were soon filled with new cases – many of them young African children, presumably none of whom had been vaccinated.

But there were many young expatriate men as well. Several young policemen were brought in, in various stages of paralysis. One was completely unconscious and totally inert for several days before suddenly recovering completely. Others were not so lucky and had varying degrees of residual paralysis, especially of limbs, even after the period of recovery had long passed. Doctors and nurses were working virtually round the clock, with little or no rest or respite.

My fevers now became recurrent and exhausting and didn't respond to the standard anti-typhus therapy. The beautifully cooked meals brought before me evoked no vestige of appetite and I changed rapidly from 'trencherman' to 'hunger-striker'! Analysis of blood samples sent to Professor Gear the South African Medical Research Centre at Ondersterpoort eventually came up with a diagnosis of West Nile virus, transmitted by mosquitoes from birds and causing a self-limiting infection with high dengue-like fevers.

Arthropod-borne viruses were then a largely unclassified group. The infection eventually faded away spontaneously, but for some years I experienced occasional and unexplained fevers and sweats and wondered if this wasn't 'my old friend' gently reminding me of times past!

It was here in the IDH that I met two very remarkable people; one was a beautiful blonde and highly efficient nurse (whom I was fortunate enough eventually to marry); the other was Ian Bompas – a young man who, injured and totally paralysed from the neck down with poliomyelitis, spent most of his time in an iron lung. With his infectious good humour Ian was the 'darling' of the IDH staff. In addition to being a very fine chess player, Ian taught himself to paint with the brush held in his mouth and became, or continued to be, a very fine artist. His most amazing accomplishment was to teach himself to 'frog-breathe' – constantly sipping and swallowing air. This allowed him to escape from the iron lung and enjoy being taken out on visits to the local Nairobi National Game Park in a motor caravan adapted for wheel-chair use. When his parents decided to move down south to South Africa, Ian created yet another record by frog-breathing throughout the entire journey by air from Nairobi to Jo'burg. My wife and I still cherish a beautiful Kenya coastal scene which Ian painted for us as a wedding present.

Another very sad and notable arrival at the IDH at this time was another Ian – Ian Pritchard. He had been a member of the Kenya police and having been brought up with the Kikuyu could speak their language fluently. At the time of the Mau Mau uprising Ian and his colleague, dressed as Mau Mau and smeared in mutton fat, joined up with, and captured, several members of different Mau Mau gangs that were living in the forests of Mt. Kenya. Later when normal peace was restored Ian, an expert water skier, had set up his own water sports and sub-aqua centre near to Malindi on the coast north of Mombasa. His favourite pastime was to swim into the large caves under the reef studying the huge groupers and other fish that sheltered there. Sadly, while testing some new water skis, he fell and fractured his spine making him immobile, similar to Ian Bompas, but still able to breathe without a respirator. Later his friends would tow him down into the caves under the reef to see again the huge fishes that he had earlier swum with.

My new partner and I now planned a sight-seeing trip to Uganda and duly set forth up the great north road. We slept in the car the first night in a car park in Jinja. Next morning we moved up to see the majestic outpouring of the 'White Nile' through the sluices of the new Owen Falls Dam – a fitting memorial to Speke and Grant, the first expatriates to reach the then Ripon Falls, and whose commemorative plaque now lies beneath the rushing waters of this famous river. We took the road north to Masindi and Butiaba passing through some very frightening grass fires. Although these had policemen standing guard at both ends, to advise motorists to close all windows, not to stop under any circumstances and roughly for how long the thick smoke and flames persisted. Once inside visibility was virtually nil and the roadside flames far too close for comfort; to have left the car would have been suicidal.

The Victoria Nile has its source in Lake Victoria (Nyanza) and flows westwards into Lake Albert. On our way to stay at the Paraa Lodge across the river in the Murchison Falls National Park, we reached the ferry at the crossing point in time to see it already under way. Unfortunately this was the last ferry that day and we were stuck. It was very hot and humid and there were no buildings of any kind at the ferry where we could find shelter. However, a few minutes earlier, about two or three miles back down the road, we had passed through a low-lying swampy area with a small road construction camp where a new bridge was being built to ease crossing in the rainy season. Unfortunately this seemed to suit the elephants which had assembled in the area in considerable numbers. We drove back and went up to the three metal Portacabin huts, which were surrounded by huge mounds of road chippings, gravel, sand and concrete blocks. The engineer and his wife, a young Austrian couple, seemed happy to offer us overnight accommodation, probably pleased to have someone to talk to. We added what was left of our provisions and drinks to the kitchen store and enjoyed the rest of the evening chatting over ice-cold beers.

When bed-time approached our hosts explained the safety procedures for using the 'loo' – a deep pit latrine in yet another Portacabin, sited for obvious reasons some thirty to forty yards from the house across open ground. By the back door was a large pile of gravel and we could see another similar pile outside the loo door. By the time it was dark, and in response to diuretic insistence we stepped outside to head for the loo only to find half a dozen elephants blocking the path – half way across; at first sight a 'no-go' situation!

But again our hosts had the answer – a handful of gravel was hurled up into the air to fall on and frighten the animals which, duly alarmed, moved away temporarily allowing you to nip smartly across and into the comparative sanctuary of the portacabin. The trick was now to get back again the same way – hence the pile of gravel chippings by the loo door. It worked well enough but was more than a little scarey and certainly speeded things up a bit. Being travel weary we fell asleep easily enough but the pièce de résistance was yet to come. We were rudely awakened when, sometime later, one large elephant began rubbing himself against our Portacabin bedroom, while another one was pulling mouthfuls of straw from the roof. The basso profundo rumblings of the adult elephant's digestive system are audible over quite large distances; when only a few feet away they were both deafening and frightening and we could only lie there and hope that, with the memories for which they are renowned, they would soon recollect better fare and feeding grounds elsewhere!

Fortunately, due to a combination of general fatigue and the soporific rockings of the Portacabin hut by the itching elephant, we finally fell deeply asleep and, next morning, woke early. We thanked our hosts and drove back to the Nile ferry. This was a small stern-wheeler which chugged steadily across this great river – probably knowing its way there and back blindfolded – while the helmsman was sitting up on the stern rail playing an 'African piano' with his two thumbs while nonchalantly steering with one foot on the tiller. The regular 'plinka-plonka-plink' of the metal strips provided a musical background both pleasing and totally in harmony with the occasion. Whilst it may not have gone down too well in the world's concert halls no classical concerto or symphony could have been better suited to the occasion than this simple home-made contraption in the hands of its master.

At Paraa Lodge in the Murchison Falls National Park, on the opposite bank, we were allocated a large tent mounted over a circular concrete plinth. The mosquito-netted beds were comfortable and spotlessly clean as were all the other facilities. We were warned not to leave any of the car windows even partially open. A few weeks earlier a young German couple had arrived in a Volkswagen 'Beetle', with a huge stalk of bananas on the back seat – and forgot to close the rear windows. A large bull elephant browsing nearby was drawn to investigate the attractive smell but, being frustrated by its failure to lift the bananas out, lifted the car bodily on its tusks and smashed it down several times on the ground. What was left of it was still there, just off the road to where it had been pushed.

We hired a Park Ranger and drove round to the top of the famous Murchison Falls – where this mighty Nile river plunges through a 14 ft wide gap in the rock and falls some 400 ft in a series of spectacular cascades down to the level of Lake Albert at Fajao – joining the lake proper some 16 miles further down river. The Falls have a wooden bridge spanning the cataract where you can stand with the whole of the Nile roaring and plunging away down the gorge only a very short distance below your feet. From Fajao open-sided motor launches owned by the Park Authority take visitors the mile or so up to the bottom of the falls, the banks on both sides being adorned with many resting crocodiles, most with their mouths wide open (dentists especially welcomed!) and various other animals coming to drink. There were several herds of elephants, mostly with young running about and getting tangled up between the legs of the adults but gently shepherded out of harm's way with an occasional caressing nudge from the maternal trunk.

To witness such delicacy of touch and gentleness in one so huge and powerful was very impressive. The numbers of crocodiles and hippos in this particular district are said to be 'beyond credence' and certainly we saw plenty of both.

We later drove along the eastern shores of Lake Albert to Butiaba where we stopped for a snack and a paddle in the chilly waters of the lake. Then on down towards Fort Portal where we put up the tent beside the car almost at the feet of the mighty Ruwenzoris – the fabulous 'Mountains of the Moon' which the Alexandrian astronomer and geographer Claudius Ptolemy (AD 90 – 168) considered was the source of the Nile.

Although early morning mist at first prevented any view; when it lifted, an hour or so later, this beautiful snow-capped range appeared in all its glory. We travelled on down again to the little Lake George by the Kazinga Channel. Although its water is reportedly fresh and almost potable we declined to put it to the test – especially on seeing a huge decaying hippo, belly up in the water, being torn to pieces by vultures; but it was a wonderful place for birds of all kinds. We now took the ferry down the Kazinga Channel to Lake Edward, from which the Semliki River runs north, through the Parc National Albert and the home of the pigmies in the Semliki Firest. Ultimately it joins forces, at Khartoum, with the Blue Nile coming down from the Highlands of Ethiopia – to irrigate vast tracts of Egypt, via the great Aswan Dam, on its way to Cairo, Port Said and the Mediterranean Sea.

By now our time was running short so reluctantly we turned for home via Mbarara, Kampala and Jinja, travelling round the northern shores of Lake Victoria (Nyanza) which fifty years earlier had witnessed a devastating (*Trypanosoma gambiense*) sleeping sickness epidemic, during which some 250,000 people had died. It was eventually brought under control by the unilateral action of the then Governor, Sir Hesketh Bell, who, of his own volition, authorised the wholesale movement of the villages, along the coastal fringe, further inland, away from the tsetse-infested shoreline vegetation – an action for which he was later unfairly castigated, for his timely action certainly ended the epidemic and saved many hundreds of lives.

Soon after my arrival in Kenya I had been offered accommodation with friends at Langata. Nick and his wife Monica Costa were cousins of Peter Hall with whom I had shared a cabin on the ship coming out. The house was a large wooden structure built up, off the ground, on brick piers. It had a huge shady verandah and wide steps leading out on to a large and attractive garden. Being so close to the Nairobi National Game Park it was open house at night to several different wild animal species. Hyaenas and sometimes honey-badgers (ratels) came to inspect the waste bins and occasionally we heard the sawing bark of a leopard. One particularly unwanted visitor in many Nairobi gardens was the puff-adder – a heavy sluggish and highly poisonous snake. Most snakes are sensitive to vibrations and tend to move away as one approaches, often without your seeing them at all. But, although the puff-adder is a slow mover over the ground, it strikes with lightning rapidity when roused. Often found lying in thick grass it is a constant threat to the unwary – especially to young children who will often, in their excitement, and without thinking, chase a ball into the long grass. My only close brush with this particular danger came early one Sunday morning. The previous day I had been doing a top overhaul on the engine of my little Fiat 500 'Topolino' – decoking and grinding the valves. Being unable to reassemble it completely before dark, I had put the remaining parts into a large cardboard box which I placed at the back of the verandah away from any risk of rain. Waking on this lovely sunny Sunday morning I decided to try to finish the work on the car before breakfast. I pulled the box away from the wall and stooped to lift it up to carry it outside. As I did so I heard a rustling sound and a huge puff adder rose up and, as I drew back (somewhat smartly it must be said) it immediately struck at my unprotected arm – fortunately missing me by inches. It was a very sobering experience.

A few weeks later, and wanting to take a closer look at the mighty Mt. Kilimanjaro, we decided to drive down over one sunny week-end. The tarmac road runs from Nairobi down via Athi River to the Kenya/Tanzania border some 120 miles away. We signed the book at the Namanga customs post at the border before passing the beautiful and shapely Mt. Longido (8,577ft) where the track turns off to the famous Amboseli Game Reserve. It continues down the 'Twining Highway' to the dusty but very pleasant town of Arusha – overlooked by the symmetrical volcanic cone of Mt. Meru. In the centre of town outside the New Arusha Hotel is a large sign by a huge tree in the forecourt, announcing that this hotel is exactly half-way between the Cape and Cairo. As luck would have it the clouds were right down almost to ground level and 'Kili' completely invisible. Driving back in the dark, with the others sound asleep in the back and myself fighting the soporific effect of looking only at the ribbon of tarmac lit by the headlights, I was suddenly jerked into full consciousness by the sight of a large pale brown barrier completely blocking the road ahead. The sharp braking and sudden fall in the engine note woke the sleepers. "Are we home yet?" and "What's the matter?" And answer came there none – for none was needed; by this time, the nine or ten lions and lionessess that had been stretched comfortably across the road enjoying the residual warmth of the tarmac, had risen and come to investigate the intruders that had so unceremoniously interrupted their evening snooze. They came padding up to us and some began rubbing themselves against the car. Happily for us they decided we were 'small beer' and with nothing more than a brief display of their very impressive dentition, they moved off slowly into bush and let us continue.

Only a few weeks later some of the doctors at the IDH spent a week camping at this same spot, near Namanga. One particularly warm night, foolishly perhaps, they decided to sleep out under the stars. On waking next morning they were somewhat startled to find themselves surrounded by the huge 'pug' marks of the lions which, during the night, had paid them a courtesy call; these were probably the same pride that we had nearly run into on our way home earlier. Although it is true that lions will not normally attack man there are many recorded instances where lions have invaded camps at night and carried off unprotected sleepers. Only once did I sleep out unprotected in game country. This was while returning from a brief visit to Dar es Salaam with two Scottish friends, Tess and Dennis Gower. Dennis, a Scottish mountaineering guide, was then a guide and instructor at the Outward Bound School at Loitokitok, on the northern slopes of Mt. Kilimanjaro; Tess, his wife, was a senior theatre sister at the Aga Khan hospital in Nairobi. We spent two or three days watching the trainees endure and gain confidence in overcoming the arduous routine and exercises. These included washing in freezing cold water at six a.m., followed by a short run before breakfast – then negotiating high-level rope exercises, treetop walk-ways, rapid slides down to ground level – as well as abseiling and roped climbing techniques. The course culminated in a climb of Mt. Kilimanjaro with a picnic and party photographs on the icy summit (Kaiser Wilhelm Spitze – later renamed Uhuru Peak – at 19,340 ft). The more experienced and with energy to spare, descended into the icy crater.

We set off in a short-wheel base Landrover down to Dar es Salaam, with its lovely and evocative name 'Haven of Peace' and its wonderful natural harbour – still the centre for considerable native shipping traffic and industry. To this day dhows continue to ply their trade from India and the Gulf States using the regular monsoon winds to drive them. They pick up mangrove bark from along the coast together with grain and copra and a considerable trade is still done with the Arabian coast. The town is situated on the shores of a palm-fringed bay and was only a small fishing village when the Germans occupied it in 1889. Seven years later it succeeded Bagamoyo ("Lay down your heart") as the capital of the then German East Africa, the name of which evoked terrible memories to the thousands of chained and exhausted slaves who passed through Bagamoyo on their way to the Zanzibar market. Both Zanzibar and Bagamoyo saw the departure and return of many explorative expeditions, most of them sponsored by the British Geographical Society of London with the aim of finding the true source of the river Nile. This was thought by many to be the 'mountains of the Moon', later identified and mapped in western Uganda. This quest attracted some of the brightest stars in the explorer's firmanent – Dr. David Livingstone, Richard Burton, Speke and Grant, Sir Samuel Baker and his Hungarian wife Florence and Henry Morton Stanley, all of whom showed tremendous patience, courage and determination and all adding considerably to the lustre of Victorian achievement.

Half-way back to Nairobi from Dar, and having left the main tarmac route, just north of Handeni the Landrover's petrol pump' gave up the ghost' leaving us completely stranded miles from anywhere useful. Necessity, normally the mother of invention, failed dismally to come up with anything helpful. We had no proper tools with which to dismantle the pump; however, a more thorough search in the bowels of the vehicle disclosed a long piece of rubber pipe and a roll of insulating tape. This finally gave us an answer. One end of the tube was taped down into the top of the carburettor and the other fed back through the front air vent on the passenger's side. It was then pushed down into a small hole made in the corner of a 4-gallon tin 'debbi' of petrol. This was then balanced precariously on the lap of the front passenger, a role which was rotated every 30 minutes. This expedient was effective but allowed only modest progress at about 25 mph; but it lasted out all the way back to Nairobi. However, we had to rest when it got dark and decided to sleep through and resume next morning. This was made easier when just before sundown we came across a village school and received permission to camp out on the football pitch. The ground sheet was spread out and, donning all our clothes, we curled up and, tired as we were, slept like logs. No mosquitoes – no lions – only tiny ants which woke us on a sunny dawn, fortunately not the dreaded 'siafu' (driver ants) which would have had us all up in a flash and doing the demented strip dance!

CHAPTER 10

Monkey Business

Field research with Prof. Garnham at the 'Bushwhackers' safari camp, Kibwezi – reed pipe opens door to Pate Island – first proof of sleeping sickness in a wild animal

At about this time Professor Garnham, Professor of Medical Protozoology at the London School of Hygiene & Tropical Medicine, was writing his 'magnum opus' – a comprehensive exposition entitled 'The Malaria Parasites' – a subject on which he was a world authority. Many, perhaps most, animals in Africa are infected with malaria-like parasites (Sub-phylum: Sporozoa), i.e. those producing massive numbers of spore-like bodies (called sporozoites) at the end of the reproductive cycle in the primary host – in this case the insect vector. One particular parasite cycle remained unresolved – that of the monkey malaria (*Hepatocystis kochi*) – with which many monkeys in the African bush are infected. Unusually only the sexual cells (gametocytes) are found in the circulating blood of the monkeys and nothing at all was known of the extrinsic parasite development cycle in the insect, since the vector had yet to be identified and studied. A minute midge (*Culicoides* species) the vector of the common worm infection (*Acanthocheilonema dirofilaria perstans* – sorry!) was highly suspect but, although many had been dissected no evidence of developing *H.kochi* parasites had been found in their salivary glands. Not very surprising, it may be thought, given that Culicoides midges are only 1-2 mm long and called, in the USA, with engaging realism, 'no-see-ums'!

It was assumed that the massive parasite multiplication phase in the insect vector would appear as small globular cysts on the outer surface of the stomach wall, protruding into the fluid-filled body cavity – in the same way as the malaria parasites of humans develop in the Anopheline mosquito. Dissecting out the salivary glands of a mosquito, to see if it is ready to transmit malaria to man, may seem something of a 'labour of Hercules': dissecting out the salivary glands of a 1mm long Culicoides midge more the province of the stand-up comedian! However, with proper tools and a little practice such dissections are comparatively easy to do. Donald Minter, Dr. Heisch and I each dissected many hundreds of these tiny midges – rupturing the pale glands in a small drop of saline solution and examining them under the microscope for the presence of the pale, greenish refractive eel-like sporozoites; but not one was positive. To assist this study the logical approach was first to identify monkeys infected with this parasites; secondly to expose these as 'sentinel bait' in a natural *Culicoides* location and, lastly, to catch all the insects coming to feed on them and, after a brief holding period to allow any latent infection to develop, to dissect and examine them.

Platforms were built at various heights in the tree canopy on which the caged monkeys would be placed. Two areas were chosen initially, one in the Ngong forest just north of Nairobi: the other inside the Nairobi National Game Park. Ladders and handrails were put in place with fixed ropes to assist the less agile climbers. Donald, the entomologist, brought his natural inventive ability to bear and designed an ingenious suction trap with a special timing device wired up to a neatly modified alarm clock. The minute hand made regular contact for two minutes in every five. The trap had a small attached bottle into which the insects were sucked and kept for later dissection. It worked beautifully for several weeks without a single failure.

But the Ngong venue proved sadly unproductive and activities were soon transferred into the Nairobi National Park. Both expatriate and local staff took it in turns to monitor the sentinel monkeys and traps on a 'two on – four off' basis. This was pleasant enough during the day but at night the quarter of a mile walk from the tented camp (itself not entirely immune to inspection by the larger predators!) to the catching area, armed only with flashlights and an over-active imagination, could be little scary. There had been several instances where National Park staff, riding to work on their bicycles, had challenging encounters with mischievous adolescent lions. The few biting midges caught there were identified as harmless *Lasiohelia* species and all were negative.

It was finally decided to move the study to a warmer, lower location (Nairobi is a little under 5000ft above mean sea level) one where *H.kochi* infections in monkeys are common. At this stage Professor Garnham came out from London to lead the investigation team. The place chosen was 'Bushwhackers' – a safari camp near Kibwezi owned and run by a former big-game hunter and his wife; Hugh and Jane Stanton; but like many other hunters he had forsaken the killing of animals and had taken to conserving and photographing them.

Unlike many present-day camps, catering for the self-indulgent, with their blue swimming pools, colour TV and constant satellite communications, Bushwhackers had only basic but very adequate facilities. The thatched huts had sand floors, simple wooden furniture, a large Dietz kerosene lantern for subdued lighting, a wash-stand with jug and water for ablutions and a communal outside 'loo' block. If diuretically disturbed at night remember always to take a strong torch and have something on your feet, preferably gum-boots, just in case. But don't forget to turn them upside down and knock them well first, to dislodge any itinerant scorpions that may have decided to move in and claim settler's rights!

Feeding too was communal and, despite a slightly less extensive and sophisticated menu, excellent. Two important attractions were the close proximity of the Athi river to which, on both banks, many different animal species came down to drink and the elephants also to wash and wallow: the other was a large tree platform. This had been built in a huge tree and had a thatched roof, wooden floor and a low protective wall. It overlooked a large and well-patronised salt-lick which attracted a wide variety of wild-life (other than ourselves) – rhino and calf, buffalo, lions, warthogs (usually en famille all running about with tails erect) and many of the larger antelopes – especially kudu and eland. Access was via a strong rope ladder which was hauled up and secured beyond the reach of aspiring simian and feline alpinists! Bed rolls, blankets, flasks of hot coffee, sandwiches and binoculars were provided. Once safely established the supply truck drove off back to the camp. Lying there quietly in the pale moonlight one had a wonderful grand-stand view of the animals as they came and went, some quietly with stealth ever ready for danger: others with much noisy grunting and seeming arrogance.

For the scientific programme two large trees were chosen some distance from the camp; one in thickish bush: the other on the bank of the Athi river. Three platforms were built in each at approximately 12, 25 and 40 ft levels with secure rope-ways and ladders between for easy and safe access and one caged monkey was placed on each. Continuous catches were made by day and by night – each infected 'sentinel' monkey being watched and fed by the pair of staff members on duty. We all worked in shifts round the clock. One morning driving down to the tree site before dawn to start my shift, in the headlights I could see that the lower two platforms were unoccupied and all 6 staff members were huddled together on the top platform. As I approached they shouted down "Angalia sana, Bwana Roy, ipo simba karibu chini – unaweza kumsikia (Watch out – there's a lion about down there – you can hear him). When I switched off the Landrover engine I could hear a repeated growling sound, just below where I was standing; but it sounded more like the sawing grunt of a leopard. A gradual brightening of the eastern sky announced the imminent arrival of dawn and, as the light grew stronger, a dark shape could be seen in the river about 10 yards from the foot of the tree. Binoculars showed it to be a very large baboon – up to its chest in the water, clearly immobile and almost certainly injured.

Having put the research programme back on the rails and with a much relieved staff at their proper stations again, I drove back to camp and roused Dr. George Nelson. He brought his rifle and quickly put the baboon out of its misery with a bullet through the head. The lads then waded in and brought it to the bank where, on examination, it was found to have a broken back, probably sustained from having fallen from the tree. Although several hundred midges, that had fed on the infected monkeys, were caught and, after an appropriate holding period, dissected, no sign of the monkey malaria parasites were seen. The final piece of this particular puzzle was later fitted into place back at the 'London School'. Prof took some of the preserved insects back with him and his technician Percy Nesbitt, of his own initiative, embedded some in wax and cut serial longitudinal and sagital sections of them. When these were later stained, mounted on a glass slide and examined under the microscope the 'missing' developing stages of the parasite could clearly be seen – not attached to the gut as expected, but in spaces in the head. *Culicoides adersi* was then finally confirmed as one vector of monkey malaria, in all probability the main one. Prof. Garnham was able to complete its life cycle in his book – truly a magnum opus!

Another cheerful little chap at Bushwhackers was a tame bush-baby (Night-ape – or small tree-climbing lemur *Galago senegalensis*). These are small furry ape-like creatures with large eyes, ears and sticky paws – all very useful for leaping about in trees at night. One evening we were all sitting round in the lounge enjoying a night-cap when a huge tarantuloid spider ran across the floor. Like a bolt from the blue the galago swept down on to it from his perch on the open rafters. In a flash it had grabbed the spider, made an equally prodigious leap on to a tall sideboard where it proceeded to devour it with (and without) relish, bits of legs and body falling down from above! It later did the rounds of the company perching on willing shoulders and shamelessly sipping any drinks offered to it (clearly a habit to which it had become accustomed). The number of willing shoulders fell away markedly when host Hugh Stanton explained that all bush-babies and galagoes (night apes) retain the stickiness of their paws by urinating on them!.

During much of this time the other DIBD unit in Kisumu was working on onchocerciasis (river blindness) and sleeping sickness (African human trypanosomiasis) around Lake Victoria and the Nile and finally succeeded in eradicating the vector flies (*Simulium neavei*); interestingly the larvae had been found earlier (by Prof. Garnham) developing on the backs of the fresh-water-crabs in the fast-flowing rivers. The Mombasa-based unit was meanwhile concentrating mostly on trying to control malaria and Bancroftian filariasis (elephantiasis) at the coast.

Several areas of Kenya are infested with tsetse flies; the Mara river area at the north of the end of the famous Serengeti plain, now so well known and widely visited by many wild-life safari visitors to what is now the Masai-Mara Game Reserve, was completely closed to visitors during the 1939-1945 war. The first Game Warden that went into that area after the war quickly became infected with sleeping sickness, which suggested strongly that the infection must have come from the wild animals. It had long been assumed, but never proven, that man only becomes infected when he intrudes upon the natural cycle of the parasites (trypanosomes) circulating between the game animal hosts and the tsetse fly vectors.

Dr. Heisch immediately initiated a programme of research aimed at proving that the game animals were in fact the natural reservoir of infection for this disease. He first arranged a number of volunteers willing to be injected with freshly drawn blood from wild animals in which the typical trypanosomes were present. These were Dr. Heisch himself, Charles Guggisberg (the huge Swiss bearded mammalologist), Donald Minter and his wife Celia, and myself. As mentioned earlier meanwhile Jimmy McMahon and Barney Highton in Kisumu were making excellent progress in what turned out to be the complete eradication of the *Simulium neavei* fly that was breeding in the fast-flowing streams. River blindness is a particularly unpleasant disease, the thin wire-like worms form tight nodules from which their infective microfilariae offspring migrate in their thousands into the skin, from which they are picked up by the Simulium fly when it bites to take blood. These microfilariae, carried in the blood, also migrate to the eyes where they cause ocular opacities and irreparable damage to the optic nerve – i,e, river blindness. The Simulium breed in fast flowing-rivers for the oxygen they need and it is only by dosing all rivers and subsidiary streams (with 'Abate' granules) that their eradication was eventually achieved. After their success with the Simulium control measures

Jimmy and Barney began sampling game animals in the sleeping sickness areas along the lakeshore, north of the Kavirondo Gulf. The blood from one bushbuck, shot in the Utonga Ridge area of the Sakwa peninsular, was found to have trypanosomes of the *Trypanosoma brucei* group – to which the human-infective forms belong. A sample of this blood was immediately sent down in a cold box to Nairobi for testing in the first human volunteer. Since Dr. Heisch happened to be attending a medical conference in Lisbon at the time, Charlie Guggisberg received the first injection in his forearm and a bed was made ready for him in the nearby Kenyatta Hospital. The inoculation site quickly became greatly swollen and inflamed (typical of the infected tsetse-bite 'chancre') and his temperature shot up to nearly 105 degrees. Although he insisted on trying to walk along the verandah and down the stairs, he collapsed and was quickly put into an ambulance and taken to the waiting bed. A small drop of the blood, taken from him later, showed plenty of the highly motile parasites kicking about among the blood cells – the rest of the sample was frozen in liquid nitrogen for storage and subsequent exhaustive examination. Following standard treatment with intravenous Suramin sodium (Antrypol) Guggie made a normal recovery and was soon up and about again. The news of this final proof, of the positive role of some game animals in the sleeping sickness cycle, was telegraphed to Dr. Heisch in Lisbon, where he was able to make the appropriate announcement of this major advance in Sleeping Sickness epidemiology – no doubt to great applause!

Having achieved the research objective at the first attempt no more volunteer injections were needed. By this time Dr. George Nelson, who was working on worm-infections with Dr. Chris Teasdale, had received information of a serious outbreak of trichinosis in the Mt. Kenya area. With the ending of the Mau Mau crisis the authorities made a concession to the understandable land hunger of the Kikuyu tribe by allowing some encroachment into the thickly wooded southern slopes of the Mt. Kenya massif. It appears that a party of hunters had gone up into the forest and had seen and killed a giant forest hog (*Potamochoerus porcus*). Much of it they brought back to the villages but, such is the typical African meat hunger, they ate some of it raw on the spot. Sadly for them, this animal was very heavily infected with the coiled-watch-spring larval worms (*Trichinella spiralis*) which were encysted in the striated muscle tissue of the diaphragm, tongue, muscles of the jaw, eye and rib cage. These larvae are shed by the adult female worms living in the small intestine and are carried in the blood-stream to the tissues. The hunting party returned to their villages very sick indeed after their impromptu and ill-advised feast but although, with immediate hospital treatment, most survived, some of them died of the infection. Pieces of the diaphragm of the infected animal were squeezed between two glass slides in a special 'compressorium' and were found to contain the highest number of the coiled 'watch-spring' larvae ever recorded – over 2,000 per gram.

George Nelson mounted a research study and we set up camp at Kangaita, just below the forest edge – a few miles north of Kerugoya (Pl.12). Box traps were set up in the forest and blood samples taken from all animals caught – mostly mongooses and genet cats. Checking the traps in the early morning was exciting for, at this altitude (9,000 ft) it was very cold and misty and the paths through the forest, though just wide enough for the Landrover, had few turning places to avoid the many elephants and buffaloes there. The roof-top spotlight was a boon, both for checking fallen trap doors and also detecting the large grey figures moving among the trees; with no place to turn quietly, retreating (very difficult in the dark) or switching off the engine and sitting very quietly normally avoided further trouble. In temperate zones infections with *Trichinella* occur from eating under-cooked pork or pork sausages (when ordering – play safe and ask to have them charred!). In the Arctic bears, wolves, foxes, mink. walruses and seals are all involved and some expedition members *in extremis* have died from eating polar bear meat containing *Trichinella* larvae.

With its very close links with the London School of Hygiene & Tropical Medicine the DIBD regularly had visits from 'School' academic and teaching staff. Prof. Buckley (Helminthology) joined us for a month's visit to study the mosquito-borne filarial infections (elephantiasis or 'big leg') which are very common along the East African coast. During a brief (but very enjoyable) stay at the Blue Marlin hotel in Malindi, Prof gave a very impressive demonstration of the 'pacific crawl' – by swimming quite strongly out through the considerable and breaking surf. A very quiet and modest man he was also a very accomplished glider pilot and had played international rugby football for Ireland. Leaving the delightful flesh pots of Malindi we headed north and turned back inland at the lower reaches of the Tana River. Prof. and George Nelson took the Landrover round while we loaded the remaining equipment and a goodly pile of ripe mangoes into canoes (Pl.13) and were paddled up in some style from Golbanti as far as Ngau. Here we were comfortably accommodated close to the hospital in an old German mission house. This had a large flat roof on which we sat out enjoying the evening cold beer and listening to Prof recounting some of his bush experiences in many different parts of the world. Sadly, not long after returning to England, he died as a result of complications resulting from the many times he had infected himself experimentally with different tropical parasitic worms. It was while loading up the canoes in readiness for our return trip down river that I heard some singing and walked across to the small primary school. I stood by an open window and listened, fascinated, at the children practising their Christmas carols. Africans have a wonderful sense of rhythm and harmony and this impromptu 'concert' on the morning of our departure was particularly beautiful – one to remember and cherish.

Once back in Malindi, Dr. Heisch joined us and accompanied by George Nelson and Prof. Buckley went on to Pate Island just beyond Lamu, which earlier had been a rival to Mombasa as a trading post for gold, ivory, spice and slaves. Lamu was once a Persian colony on the mouth of the Tana River and is still a port of call for coastal and Persian Gulf vessels. The great houses of its former Arab merchants have since fallen into decay but the prosperity of Lamu, which fell into decline with the cessation of the slave trade, has show signs of revival in recent years; the building of dhows there is still a considerable industry.

On Pate island a different type of filarial worm infection had been found earlier. This had been named *Brugia patei* by Prof. Buckley and he now wanted more samples for teaching back at the 'School' in London. Because of the known hostility of the islanders to strangers, Dr. Heisch had wisely asked one of his most experienced animal handlers to lead the way in. Karissa Kikoi, was a small stocky fellow with a large moustache and saucy good humour. He was also one of the very few remaining musical instrument makers and came himself from one of the local tribes. The medical party marched into Pate led by Karissa playing a kind of wooden reed flute that had a blade of grass bent into two as the reed. When played it gave off a weird howling noise which made all the dogs bark; it was periodically interspersed with fierce drumming rhythms from a kind of home-made bamboo wash-board filled with small pebbles or dried peas. This was tucked under one arm and shaken vigorously and slapped with the thumb, creating an irresistible beat to accompany the strident dying cat sounds from the flute. Those villagers who didn't fall about laughing started to sway and dance to the magical rhythm – as most African can and will. The visit was a huge success and Prof. Buckley went on his way rejoicing – with overweight baggage, full of *Brugia malayi* teaching samples.

Bancroftian filariasis (elephantiasis) is a most unpleasant disease when at its worst in highly endemic areas. Constant inoculation of the infective larvae by mosquitoes over many years builds up a concentration of adult worms. These move in the blood to the lymph drainage channels, often in the legs and groin, which they often block completely. The local reaction and the physical blockage cause the massive tissue overgrowth of the legs, scrotum and groin – aptly described as elephantiasis. The infective larvae appear in the blood after dark, with maximum levels being reached in the early hours – between midnight and 2 or 3 a.m. This coincides precisely with the peak biting time of the vector mosquitoes. By day not a single microfilaria may be seen but progressively from 10 p.m. onwards their numbers in the peripheral circulation increase rapidly until about 2 a.m. when the blood is swarming with them. This pattern of behaviour is know as nocturnal periodicity and the physiological factors that underlie it, discovered by Professor Frank Hawking, are the host's circadian rhythm, the difference in oxygen tension between arterial and venous blood by day and night and by changes in body temperature and the adaptive rhythm of the parasite. Professor Hawking, a tropical parasitologist of international renown, was also father of the even more famous son Stephen – the very eminent Cambridge astrophysicist of 'black holes' fame.

Towards the end of my contract, Dr. Heisch called me into his office and told me that, despite his best efforts to obtain a Government bursary, to help me gain my University degree, he had been unsuccessful. At that time the 'winds of change' were blowing strongly across sub-Saharan Africa and a date had rightly been set for Kenya's independence. Because of this, bursaries were to be given only to those who were Kenya citizens or who had had all of their schooling in Kenya. This was the 'writing on the wall' for me – writ large. Although I had built up a useful fund of practical experience, both in the field and in the laboratory, I was still highly unqualified and, in a newly independent Kenya my future looked far from promising. But I had much to look forward to; my beautiful blonde nurse, in a moment of madness, had accepted to marry me and now, having established that tropical diseases research was to be my 'chosen career', I had decided to start climbing the academic ladder the hard way.

I bade a reluctant farewell to all members of the DIBD staff – in particular to the African staff who had taught me so much and had accepted my occasional gaffes with understanding and good humour – rightly attributing them to naivety and ignorance, with no element of ill will or arrogance. I would miss them all very much. Now, in retirement many years later, I still warm to the memory of their cheerful and ungrudging support.

CHAPTER 11

Join the W.H.O.

The Brompton Hospital, London – W.H.O. malaria team in northern Nigeria

I sailed home on the Braemar Castle from Mombasa, sad at leaving my beautiful partner and also the many friends and colleagues that had enriched my experience in such a wonderful country. I had a genuine desire to return but knew that, if it happened at all, it would be long in coming and that there was much to be done in the meantime. While the ship was sailing through the Canal a small party of us took a coach to Cairo and, after a night in a hotel, visited the Sphynx, the Pyramids and the famous Museum of Antiquities. This latter, in particular, was totally absorbing but there were far too many sarcophagi, wonderful hand-made golden ornaments and stone statues to absorb at a single visit. We rejoined the ship at Port Said. The rest of the voyage home was uneventful and the general atmosphere among the passengers bore no resemblance to the happy anticipation that had epitomised the attitude of those on the journey out. In an attempt to reach home for the New Year a few of us jumped ship at Marseilles and boarded a fast train to Calais. It left precisely on time and although travelling at great speed we were able to dine in comfort with no spilled wine or coffee and could walk down the gangway without being thrown off balance every few steps. By contrast, the train that took us from Dover to Victoria, with its pictures of Victorian bathing huts at Bognor Regis adorning the compartment, its dirty windows, hard red and black cushioned seats and much of our coffee in the saucers, underlined our return to mundane reality.

With both my parents now dead I took temporary lodging with my sister whilst I set about trying to put together the remnants of my promising career. I had to accept that, for the moment, a degree course was out of the question and that I needed to start earning some money quickly if I had any hope of supporting a wife. Although a return to the laboratories of the London School of Hygiene &

Tropical Medicine seemed at first to be the obvious choice I first needed to qualify in basic medical laboratory technology. Probably the best place for this, at that time, was in the medical laboratories of the Brompton Chest hospital in London. The standard textbook in medical laboratory technology was by a Mr. Frank Baker – the Chief Technician (Bacteriology) there; he also lectured at evening classes in Bacteriology.

The return soon after of my fiance and our wedding preceded a quick return to the sun in Cattolica on the Italian Adriatic. My new parents-in-law (''outlaws"as I called them) made room for us in their London home; our faithful VW beetle, with some 80,000 African miles on its clock, arrived home safely in the London docks and I started work at the Brompton and, once again, found myself attending evening classes. By this time, now 36 years old and still with only 3 'A' levels, I was working with 16 – 17 year-olds fresh from school. I was earning just enough to keep our heads above water. But only the fact that my wife returned to nursing, as a very busy Senior Ward Sister in the St. Helier Hospital, Carshalton, kept us from joining Davy Jones's Sub-Aqua Club!

For the first activity I was washing up glassware and preparing culture media, sharing a double-sink in the basement with Elsie. Her husband had run off and left her with a mentally sub-normal son who, now nearly adult, was causing her much concern. Despite her life of unending drudgery on little pay Elsie was invariably cheerful and always concerned with helping others with their problems – an unwitting teacher of basic philanthropy to those who thought themselves hard done by. Every Friday afternoon I queued up with the youngsters for my £9.50 which I took home to my very patient and enterprising young wife.

The compression of some 3 years of study into less than 18 months, coupled with the mind-bending rush-hour commuting to and from London, brought me close to a nervous breakdown but was successful. Shortly before receiving the final examination results for bacteriology (in which I was successful), out of the blue one morning I received a letter from the World Health Organisation H.Qs in Geneva, asking me if I would be interested in joining a newly-formed malaria research team in Northern Nigeria. On the strength of my positive reply (probably received there still warm from its ultra-rapid transit) I was summoned to Geneva for interview and medical. This gave me my first chance to see the Alps from the air, looking down on the snow-covered knife-edge ridges, the 'bergschrund' crevasses and the beautiful snow-draped mountain architecture brought back many happy memories of winter climbing days in

Scotland and in the beautiful Jotunheimen area of Norway. Flying down Lake Geneva at low level, in daylight on final approach to Cointrin Airport, provided a wonderful view of the magnificent 400 ft high 'Jet d'eau' fountain trailing its windblown curtain of spray across the lake – a fitting welcome to this lovely city.

Soon after Christmas I went back again to Geneva for briefing before flying out again with UTA to Brazzaville – the W.H.O.'s Regional Office for Africa (AFRO). As with all W.H.O. buildings this was a magnificent affair built in a 60 acres site at Djoué some 6 miles up-stream from Brazzaville. This was my first visit to francophone Africa and I immediately felt at ease in the more informal and relaxed atmosphere. I also fell in love with the local Congolese music, particularly enjoying the songs of the world-famous 'Franco'. Most of the buildings tended to be a little 'down-at-heel' and needed several licks of paint; our hotel, the Metropole, was no exception and although over-patronised by cockroaches had plenty of the excellent 'Primus' beer which more than atoned for their unwelcome presence. French expatriates believe in living life to the full and the shops want for nothing; cargo planes, arriving daily from France, were bringing in virtually everything one could wish for. The food available in the Brazzaville hotels and restaurants was excellent and reasonably priced.

The Regional Office itself was modern and fully air conditioned, but it is sad to think that, only a few years ago during the civil strife there, the rebels completely destroyed this beautiful building – thankfully not before all W.H.O. and expatriate staff had been moved into a new Regional Office in Harare, Zimbabwe. Sadly, this country, too, has recently experienced serious political difficulties and economic decline and it must be doubtful whether, in the absence of changes for the better, the W.H.O. staff can continue to function there for very much longer. The ownership of a piece of land on which to grow one's subsistence crops, is a *sine qua non* of the average African, as it is with many of us, and freedom from tribalistic animosities coupled with a more equitable redistribution of land in many countries of sub-Saharan Africa, not only in Zimbabwe, difficult though that would be in some cases, would obviate some if not all of the unrest and political tensions.

Malaria pre-eradication teams were being formed to work in several different parts of sub-Saharan Africa. I was assigned to one in Sokoto Province, northern Nigeria, led by Dr. Peter Kim – a tall, pleasant and personable malariologist from South Korea. We were first sent to the W.H.O. Malaria Eradication Training Centre based in the grounds of the West African Medical Research Unit at Yaba, in Lagos. Here some

20 doctors of different nationalities were training as malariologists – we joined them for lectures and some practical sessions but, for the most part, were working directly with Gerald Shute, the senior W.H.O. technician in the laboratories. To gain as much experience as possible in a short space of time we visited several of the outlying villages to examine and treat the people. The clinics run by the METC Director, Dr. Mac Dowling, were very popular and villagers came from miles around when the word got out that we were coming. These field activities were both very interesting and satisfying, since most of those attending were quickly diagnosed and treated at these clinics. The children too were carefully examined and treated for a wide range of conditions; some had huge suppurating ulcers, others were clearly malnourished, almost all were anaemic and had large spleens typical of early malaria infections. The very young children were each given a sweet, kindly supplied in large sacks, gratis, by a local firm, which put an immediate stop to the crying and made the all-important blood sampling and spleen palpation possible. Fear is infectious and a crying child will quickly set all the other children crying, making any further examinations almost impossible.

Lagos is a thrusting city – a human ant's nest – seething with life of all kinds. The wide variety of people and dress is matched by the rich variety of vehicles that block all roads. There are saloons in many gleaming colours, huge lorries old and new and the buses, mostly decrepit, sadly sagging badly after many years of overloading, neglect and abuse, but still grinding along, steam pouring from radiators and with excess passengers still clinging like bunches of grapes from invisible handholds. All of these were interspersed with locust-like swarms of motor-bikes, scooters and mopeds – many using the pavements to avoid the congested roads and blaring their horns at any misguided pedestrians having the temerity to get in their way!

The natural ebullience and good-natured philosophy of the Nigerians is well reflected in the flamboyant titles of the many ubiquitous 'Mammy Wagons' – with names like "Sea Never Dry" – "Thy Time is Best O Lord" – "No Condition Permanent"; also, within a week of the inaugural flight of the new VC10 to Kano from London, 'VC 11'!

Whilst in Lagos two new pieces of traffic legislation were passed; firstly, to ease the general traffic congestion, one allowed vehicles with even last numbers to use the roads on Mondays, Wednesdays and Fridays: those with odd last numbers on Tuesdays, Thursdays and Saturdays – with the usual free-for-all on Sundays. The second law made mandatory the wearing of safety crash helmets by all motor cyclists and mopeds users. These metaphorically threw down a political gauntlet that the local man-in-the-street, with his love of a challenge to his innate ingenuity, was only too happy to pick up.

Within a few days the back-street artisans were doing a roaring business – some quickly modifying the number plates with interchangeable last digits painted on a small hinged flap. Others, more artistic, devoted themselves to the making of safety crash helmet from gourds. These were genuine works of art and a joy to behold – painted in shiny colours with racy emblems, black-and-white checkerboard bands and snug chin-straps and plastic goggles they were almost impossible to distinguish from the genuine article. Almost certainly their rapid appearance indicated many back-street 'pavement industries' working overtime and doubtless fully engaged in a very lucrative business.

But the Lagos traffic police weren't easily fooled and quickly found a sure and simple way to detect the fraud and catch the offenders. Riders were stopped at random and made to remove their helmets. These were then placed on the pavement or road and jumped on by the heavily booted policemen. The calabash versions disintegrated immediately into many pieces and a cloud of dust, whereupon the offender would be made to do skip-jumps, press-ups or jogging-on-the-spot for a few minutes – much to the delight of the rapidly gathering crowd of amused and applauding onlookers – pleased at the prospect of some free light entertainment!

The last month of the W.H.O. malaria training course was destined to be spent doing practical field work in the north of Nigeria – at Birnin Kebbi, the home of the Nigerian Government's Mass Malaria Control Campaign (MMCC). Since this was where I had been assigned to work, and since the first of our vehicles (a Peugeot 404 estate-car) had recently arrived in the Lagos docks, I was given permission to drive it up. This was fortunate for, by then, my wife and 6-month old baby girl had just arrived from the UK and we were able to travel the 750 miles to Birnin Kebbi with our baggage in comparative comfort.

The road north from Lagos, at least as far as Ibadan, is notoriously dangerous. For the first 10 miles or so it crosses many creeks, the iron bridges for which are (or were then) incomprehensibly narrow – wide enough for one vehicle only. The number of wrecked cars and lorries adorning the approaches on both sides bore tacit witness to the many losers of the 'first across' contests. One almost new sky-blue Peugeot 404 saloon, the driver realising too late that the oncoming vehicle was already on the bridge, was bent almost in half around a sturdy tree at the roadside. One particular sad sight was that of a huge freight lorry with an equally huge trailer which had left the road and plunged down a steep embankment to finish upside down and half submerged in the creek. It was full of long-horned cattle, probably en route for the abbatoir; those that had survived the impact and drowning were still bellowing pitifully.

The journey up to Birnin Kebbi, via Ibadan and with an overnight stop in the Ilorin Government resthouse (neat, beautifully kept and comfortable) was successful. Having crossed the Niger River on the Jabba bridge, we moved on to Kontagora and so to BK. Despite the very dry heat (40 degrees Centigrade) it was a relief to escape the stifling humidity of Lagos. Birnin Kebbi is a small town some ninety-five miles south of Sokoto and the home of the Emir of Gwandu. Its few shops had only tinned food, packets of biscuits, matches, safety pins and tins of kerosene – but no fresh food of any kind. The open-air market in Birnin Kebbi was huge and kept us supplied with chickens and sometimes with pieces of beef and goat meat. Apart from the very occasional rationed donations of greenstuff from the Emir's garden, all fruit and vegetables had to be bought either in Sokoto or more reliably from Kano or Kaduna some 450 miles away. For this we were lucky in buying a virtually new Peugeot 403 station wagon from an English agricultural scientist who had just been offered a job with a UN organisation in a different country.

We had a pleasant fully-screened house with an outside 'cage' for sleeping in the hot season. This had a stout roof and was fully screened all round. The daytime temperatures varied between 110 and 115 degrees Fahrenheit but fell to below 100 at night. We were soon into the Harmattan season which was very misty and dull, like a typical winter's day in Europe but it was still very warm during the day. At night the cold katabatic wind flowed down from the Sahara and was named the 'doctor', from the relief it brought from the daily heat. Atmospheric humidity fell right off the clock and some pieces of furniture would suddenly split right across with a loud crack like a pistol shot. We all took to putting generous dollops of olive oil into the bath water to freshen the skin.

The rain when it came was sudden and violent, wind-driven, horizontal and usually preceded by a dark blue-brown curtain of wind-blown dust. Visibility in the storm was virtually nil; only the almost perpetual lightning flashes making it possible to drive at a slow walking pace. There were magnificent cumulo-nimbus thunder clouds with their huge wind-blown anvils and often line squalls, one of which uprooted the well anchored Flying Doctor plane in Gusau, sending it cartwheeling across the aerodrome where it came to rest, upside down among the trees.

With a very low water table the wells were 80-90 ft deep and the household's 'Aquarius' spent much time in hauling the cold and very clean water with a plaited rope over wooden rollers using a bucket made from rubber inner tube. Water was stored in two 44 gallon drums mounted up on a plinth with space for a wood fire underneath.

The advent of the comparatively inexpensive and highly effective insecticide DDT and the therapeutic drug chloroquine made it theoretically and technically possible to eradicate malaria from the world. The caveats, and they were many and large, being feasibility under differing conditions, the need for sustained high levels of efficiency on key aspects, sufficient numbers of trained staff, both local and expatriate, that would work well with minimal supervision, variations in affordability, preparedness of collaborating countries and, not least, the absence of any inimical influencies on the efficacy of the insecticide. At the time there was no evidence of any build-up of resistance in the vector anopheline mosquitoes to DDT nor was it foreseen that, for any number of reasons, some villagers would try to avoid having their homes sprayed.

The theory, though, was excellent – when the DDT was mixed with water and sprayed on to the inner mud walls of village huts it retained its killing power of mosquitoes for up to six months – the poison being absorbed in cumulative doses through the feet of the mosquitoes landing and resting on the walls. On the strength of this, and because of the dire need to reduce the death and misery caused by this disease throughout the tropics, especially in Africa, the World Health Organisation decided to initiate a global malaria eradication programme.This was to be preceded by a pre-eradication stage, where all countries were assisted in making an accurate assessment of the nature and extent of the malaria problem in their countries and in training the extra staff needed, to bring the operational infrastructure up to the standard required and to supply new vehicles and equipment where necessary. It was certainly ambitious but was enthusiastically received in most countries – especially those such as India and Ceylon, where mosquito control activities had already achieved a high level of success in significantly reducing both mortality and morbidity rates due to this disease; many large areas being virtually free from malaria for the first time ever.

Technically the project (Nigeria 32) was a W.H.O. Malaria Pre-eradication Programme which, although closely linked with the existing Government's Mass Malaria Control Campaign (MMCC) at Birnin Kebbi, also had a much larger remit – covering the whole of northern Nigeria – some 200,000 sq miles. This latter was merely for the collection and analysis of malaria data (both parasitological and entomological) on which could be based a general eradication strategy. The research area based on Birnin Kebbi covered some 750,000 people among which the malaria incidence/transmission had been drastically reduced over a number of years, but never completely interrupted.

The theory of malaria eradication was simple enough and based on the very sound premise that if mosquitoes come to bite and afterwards, when fully fed with blood, prefer to fly up and rest on the walls of the hut, the insecticide would kill them within the 12-14 days needed for the malaria parasites, taken up when feeding on a positive sleeper, to develop and produce the many thousands of infective spores that, injected with the saliva into a new clean host, would initiate a fresh infection. When carried to the liver in the blood stream these new parasites (sporozoites) enter the scavenging (Küpfer) cells lining the blood filtration channels of the liver. Once inside they undergo massive multiplication by simple division and, when the swollen liver cells ruptures, are released back into the blood stream – this time to invade the red blood cells.

Further parasite multiplication bursts the red cell, releasing some 10-20 tiny 'signet-ring' parasite which immediately enter fresh red cells; these repeated releases of new broods of parasites into the bloodstream every 48 hours, cause the fever peaks typical of 'cerebral' (*Plasmodium falciparum*) malignant tertian malaria. Of the four species of malaria that infect man cerebral malaria is by far the most deadly. Its rate of multiplication far exceeds that of the others; but also important, it is the only species that produces a stickiness on the outer surface of the infected red cells which causes them to adhere when they touch and collide with one another in the circulating blood to form larger and larger cellular clumps. These eventually block some of the fine blood vessels in the brain, which then swell and finally rupture causing the often lethal intercranial haemhorrages typical of 'cerebral' malaria. The insecticide chosen for the malaria eradication programme was DDT – since it was cheap, comparatively safe (when properly used) and was shown to kill a wide range of insects when sprayed on to the inside walls of huts and houses as an aqueous solution containing 2.4 grams per litre. Its lethal efficiency lasted some 6 months so that only two spraying sessions were needed each year. Entomological studies had shown that the mosquitoes in the area were feeding almost entirely on humans and, after feeding, were shown to prefer resting on the inside walls of the huts and not flying outside. Thus, provided these inner walls and roofs of all huts were regularly and properly sprayed the mosquitoes would die before the completion of the parasite development cycle (twelve to fourteen days), malaria transmission would cease and those staying within the protected area would be free of malaria for the first time. Sensitivity of the adult mosquitoes to DDT was tested regularly by exposing a standard number in a plastic cone held against the inside wall of a DDT-sprayed hut.

To eliminate the existing reservoir of infection, all people were examined and those positive for malaria were given a standard curative dose of chloroquine (Pl.28). At birth every infant was registered and examined every month until twelve months old. Special surveys were made of children 2 – 14 years and a number of larger villages were examined every three months where all age groups were included. To ensure an accurate evaluation of the eradication method the protect area was itself surrounded by a large cordon sanitaire. All people going out or coming in would be examined and receive presumptive anti-malaria treatment.

We were a truly international team, with Dr. Peter Kim from Korea as team leader; our young entomologist from Thailand we never saw for, sadly, after his briefing in the African Regional Office, Brazzaville, the DC4 aeroplane bringing him up to Nigeria crashed into the 17,700ft Mt. Cameroon in thick cloud killing all on board. He was replaced by Gamal Bakri, an experienced Egyptian entomologist domiciled in Germany. The sanitarian responsible for the spraying activities was David Thomas who, with his typically Welsh sense of humour and wide experience, was able to overcome most of the difficulties that the spraying programme encountered.

CHAPTER 12

Working with W.H.O.

Probably eradicate malaria from 750,000 people in N. Nigeria – visit Cameroons – see red and convert water into wine

The malaria laboratories consisted of two long buildings, one for parasitology (Pl.14) and the other for entomology. Both had a long bench down one side with plenty of fly-screened windows. The standard W.H.O. equipment arrived and brought us good quality Olympus binocular research microscopes but an immediate difficulty was that we had no electricity to power them. The lack of good quality microscopes, that can function successfully without reliance upon generated electricity or vehicle battery power, persists still in the non-electrified rural areas of Africa (and probably in many other tropical countries also). It is sobering to reflect that 70% or more of the populations of many developing countries live in the rural areas – where malnutrition, lack of clean water, poor sanitation and a wide range of communicable diseases continue to reap a grim harvest of mortality and morbidity – especially in the very young. During the dry season the daylight was fairly constant but not really bright enough for microscopy at the high magnifications needed for detailed diagnosis. During the rainy season or the dusty Harmattan, whenever it was cloudy the light was insufficient. Having identified a good local carpenter we set him to make some large wooden screens. These were slung outside the laboratory windows on adjustable ropes and the surfaces painted white. These reflectors worked well and enabled us to make a start on the backlog of blood films needing microscopical examination. Soon afterwards however, we made six bench lamps from inverted copper trays, vehicle headlamp bulbs and 'Camping-Gas' lamp glasses. These we connected to a high capacity vehicle battery, under the bench, which was kept charged up on the project Landrovers. A boiling flask filled with a weak solution of copper sulphate and placed in front of the mirror acted as a magnifier and gave excellent lighting with a pale blue cast – ideal for malaria microscopy. Each of the six experienced microscopists, trained with the MMCC, examined a minimum of fifty blood slides a day and, since the spraying programme was so successful almost all of these were negative and thus required particularly careful examination. This was tiring work and the staff were encouraged to take a 10 minute break every hour. Some 5,000 blood-slides were examined every month.

Such was the importance of achieving complete eradication of malaria in the population and the cessation of transmission within the protected area, that every single malaria-positive slide found (and there were very few) triggered off a major epidemiological investigation aimed at showing, if possible, that the infection had, almost certainly, been acquired outside the protected zone. It was of course impossible to prove this conclusively. Running down the western side of the project area was the Rima river which, in the hot season, dried up partially to form a series of large disconnected pools. This was called the 'fadama'; where shallow it was highly fertile and was ideal for rice cultivation; in other parts it was quite deep and covered with floating weed. Since many of the local people had friends and relatives on the other side, which was outside the protected area, there were many occasions when they took a canoe across to visit them. This was often in the cool of the evening or during the night and so the risk of acquiring a malaria infection en route, or while staying in the unprotected villages on the other side, was very high.

Although mercifully few these epidemiological investigations sometimes proved extremely difficult to complete satisfactorily. One example will suffice. A young mother living in a small village bordering the fadama had a new baby which, after four or five negative monthly blood films, suddenly showed a new and severe malaria infection. Intense questioning of the mother established that the baby hadn't been away from the village since birth, implying that transmission must have occurred within the village. It seemed unshakeable. One day later, on seeing an old man sitting alone in this village, I found out that he was the girl's grandfather and, by adroit questioning, established that they had many relatives living across the fadama, that they had visited them there recently to attend a wedding and, yes, the young woman and her baby had gone with them in the canoe and had stayed there for several days and nights before returning. When later I talked with her in confidence she confessed to having a boyfriend over there and took the opportunity of her husband's business visit to Ilorin, in the south, to renew the acquaintance. It was almost certain that the child had been bitten several times whilst in the unprotected area and would have been infected there; but, again, it was sadly impossible to prove or even make it public!

Careful examination of the various activities soon showed a number of minor, but important, shortcomings. Although the insecticidal spraying of every inhabited hut was absolutely vital it was found that a number had been missed completely and the reason for this quickly became apparent. In the absence of a shiny new car in the front drive or a digital TV dish adorning the front of the hut, for many people in the Birnin Kebbi-Argungu area the tacit expression of affluence was the collection of gourds and calabash bowls – many of them beautifully and artistically decorated. These were usually stacked high and, in some huts, reached the roof, leaving little room to move and making entrance almost impossible. Thus, when the sprayman arrived with his team the owner either had to move all the gourds outside while the hut was sprayed or, if possible, and the sprayman happened at that time to be a little short of the 'ready', slip him a modest inducement to pass by without stopping. Another more valid and acceptable reason was that the irritation of the DDT stimulated the resident and protesting bedbug and flea populations to even greater activity, so disrupting the sleep of the poor occupants more than usual. This provoked some strong feelings against the spraying which the innocent spraymen had to counter; understandably they weren't always successful.

This created a major scientific problem since these unsprayed huts provided a 'safe haven' and soon the word got round among the remaining mosquito squadrons who, like their human counterparts, were always looking for safety and shelter with free and regular meals and a place to put their feet up! These huts soon became the 'place to be' – serving to maintain a localised flare-up of new cases that were difficult to find and eliminate. Man-biting mosquitoes in the area normally rested indoors after feeding and, if undisturbed, would fly out again a few days later when the blood had been fully digested, the eggs fully developed and ready for depositing on to the surface of the nearest open water. This outward flight was constantly monitored by exit traps fitted to some 'indicator' huts and was to be expected. Soon, however, freshly-fed mosquitoes, looking like tiny red currants with wings, began to appear in these exit traps which immediately sounded the alarm bells, for it indicated a possible change in mosquito behaviour; one by which the insects would avoid prolonged contact with the insecticide on the walls. It was known that the lighting of early morning fires would drive a few mosquitoes out temporarily, but this was different.

Fortunately, at a quick 'brain-storming session', Peter Kim very brightly suggested fitting inlet traps around some of the indicator huts. These were soon installed under the eaves (a small wooden cage with white gauze funnel inside to prevent them escaping. The rest of the space between roof and wall closed off with mud and old newspapers. These new traps quickly showed the presence of freshly-fed 'flying red-currant' mosquitoes and indicated clearly that, although irritated by contact with the DDT, they still retained their preference for resting indoors and would thus eventually still pick up enough sub-lethal doses to kill them before completion of the infection cycle by any developing parasites inside them.

Another major problem that threatened to jeopardise the successful interruption of malaria transmission appeared a little later, at the end of the rainy season. This was 'transhumance' – a rather grandiose word for the regular annual mass migration of the cattle-herding nomadic Fulani herdsmen from within the protected area, literally out 'to pastures new'. The more fertile areas to the south and west were all highly malarious, Once the cattle had been suitably fattened up, and the rains had started again in the north, they were trekked back again. During this time the herdsmen, free from malaria when they trekked out, had all been heavily re-infected and acted as a new reservoir of infection from which any remnants of the local Anopheline mosquito populations quickly recharged their 'infectivity batteries' to produce another crop of worrying new cases.

This particular problem was finally overcome by forming 'fire-brigade' teams – some in Landrovers, some on bicycles and others even mounted on the ubiquitous donkeys; their sole task being to identify and intercept returning itinerant Fulani herdsmen, spray their temporary dwellings (a cage of bent saplings with woven grass 'zana' mats thrown over the top) and give everyone a presumptive 4-tablet therapeutic dose (600 mg) of chloroquine. It was hard work but eventually successful.

The final problem, that contained the hidden knock-out blow, was the emergence of mosquitoes that were resistant to the DDT. Their continuing sensitivity to the insecticide was a vital part of the eradication strategy. When resistance finally appeared it virtually signalled the end of the malaria eradication dream for, despite the possibility of switching to the use of other insecticides, which were much more expensive and less practicable, there was no acceptable alternative to a return to control measures. These in turn became infinitely more difficult when, much later, resistance of the malaria parasites to the widely-used chloroquine began to appear.

This has since become a very serious global problem – one that varies from country to country so that non-immune travellers to the tropics (with the advent of 'holidays in the sun for all' these are many and growing in numbers) must ensure that they have the appropriate drugs with them at all times and carefully follow the latest informed medical advice. The most recent 'discovery' by the 'West' was that of the therapeutic value of Artemesinin (extracted from the common Artemisia plant and used successfully by the Chinese for many years to cure malaria). Once analysed in the U.S.A. it was soon synthesised and is now widely available at a time when, in some parts of the world, it is proving increasingly difficult to cure some strains of cerebral malaria.

The riverine fadama provided much relaxation and trips out in the project's small motor-boat trying to catch the elusive but very aggressive tiger fish gave good sport. Climbing the local 'mountain' – Duku Rock – was also good fun and many late-night barbeques were held on the flat summit, the track up being well lit by many small candles in brown paper bags with earth in the bottom to keep them open. The view from the top was superb and the cool breeze brought pleasant relief from the hot and humid plains below. Open air musical evenings were also popular and 'Desert Inland Discs' became a regular favourite and the strains of Bach, Beethoven, Mozart, Grieg, Sibelius, Ravel etc floated out over the warm air and attracted sizeable crowds as did the splendid refreshments and cold beers.

Our wider remit to survey the nature and extent of the malaria problem in the different ecological zones of northern Nigeria also kept us busy. Malariometric surveys carried out over the whole of northern Nigeria were largely uneventful. Sometimes the Landrovers were sent on ahead with the equipment and the scientific staff usually followed in one or other of Nigerian Airways Dakota (DC3) aircraft from the Sokoto dirt runways. Mostly we stayed in the Government rest-houses which were clean, comfortable and with good food. A large amount of valuable epidemiological data was compiled to provide the base upon which to build the future extended eradication programme. Sadly, and unbeknown to us, the aquatic developmental stages of the vector Anopheline mosquitoes (larvae and pupae) were gradually developing resistance to the organo-chlorine insecticides being used to control the insect pests in the rice multiplication schemes along the fertile banks of the fadama to the north. Unfortunately this was quickly reflected in similar resistance developing in the mosquitoes to D.D.T. But at the time we knew nothing of this tragic turn of events, being well on our way with the country-wide surveys and temporarily out of touch with base. On this occasion we drove in a small convoy, the field staff and the equipment in two kit cars, Gamal (entomologist) and I in one Landrover with Peter Kim (malariologist) and his driver in the other. Having worked our way across from Sokoto, via Kano, Kaduna and to Jos up on the cool plateau and then down to Maiduguri in the north-east, we made a quick visit to Lake Chad and went out with some local fishermen in their reed boat – the first few minutes being taken up with travelling slowly through 10 ft high reeds which blocked all views of the lake from the shore. Once clear of them the huge extent of the lake was at once apparent.

After this we turned south-west with the dirt road hugging the line of hills running along the border with the Cameroons a few miles to the east of us and reached Jalingo at dusk. Since the completion of the Jalingo area, a few days later, coincided with a two-day national holiday, Gamal and I decided to buy extra petrol and to spend the time visiting the famous Waza Game Reserve across the border in Northern Cameroon and reasonably close. Peter opted to stay in the very comfortable Government resthouse in Jalingo to write up the survey report. We had another passenger with us, one of the members of the Government malaria unit in Birnin Kebbi who had specifically asked to join us on this field trip so that he could visit his parents in Maiduguri, whom he hadn't seen for some years. He brought along his few cooking pots and a selction of his favourite condiments; he also wanted to pay his first visit to Cameroons, There was room enough for three in the vehicle so he had joined us and was overjoyed at having seen his parents and family in Maiduguri and was as excited as were we at the prospect of visiting a neighboring country for the first time.

We worked our way slowly south down a dusty road to the border crossing point, noting the rugged terrain with its towering rock faces standing guard over narrow dried up sandy river beds on one side and the sparse stunted trees and the silvery grey thatched roofs of the discrete clusters of mud huts on the other. One thing neither Gamal nor I had seen before were the pagans who live exclusively in this area of north-eastern Nigeria. Even today they are mostly naked except for bunches of leaves fore and aft and all greeted us with friendly waves and 'keyboard' grins – clearly happy folk with a simple way of life!

Having crossed the border and turned back north again we found the roads in the Cameroons were just as varied and unpredictable in surface as those in Nigeria. The notice to 'Tenez a Droite'really meant very little and most drivers wisely used whichever part of the road looked to be least destructive and pot-holed. This was easy enough for the experienced but could be more than a little daunting to the inexperienced or irresolute! These laterite roads, sometimes yellowish grey – sometimes red, give an excellent running surface when kept smooth with a huge steel blade slung beneath a huge diesel grader. When neglected however, the vibrations set up by the passing vehicles cause the laterite particles to clump together to form regular rhythmical 'washboard' corrugations which can make it difficult to keep the vehicle on the road; their only advantage being that the incessant vibrations counteract the soporific effect of long-distance driving in the heat and dust. But these roads have one other hidden menace in the rains, when they become criss-crossed with rain-wash gullies, some of them very wide and often quite deep. In addition to the clouds of acrid and choking laterite dust that fast-moving vehicles throw up in their wake, approaching vehicles pose a more serious threat, that of a shattered windscreen, by throwing up large stones or rocks for you to run into.

At first I was pleasantly surprised to see how many on-coming drivers raised their hand to the windscreen in friendly greeting while smiling broadly. This I warmly reciprocated with a wide grin of good fellowship. A little later I discovered that the free hand touching the windscreen was to brace it against any impacting stones, which we threw up as we passed; the grin of 'bonhomie' was in fact an anticipatory grimace of impending calamity!

We drove fast, correcting the minor bumps and skids with practiced and intuitive light touches on the wheel. On one particularly smooth section, while travelling at speed, we came up a sudden rise and, reaching the crest, were greeted with a beautifully wide vista of sun-scorched scrub-land, colorful rocky outcrops and hazy distant hills. Equally wide, and stretching from one side of the road to the other, was a very large rain-wash gully – a yard or more in width and more than a foot deep. With only a few milliseconds of warning it was impossible to miss. The effect was almost total catastrophy. We hit with a terrifying crash and pandemonium broke loose – together with all the unstrapped luggage – pots and pans, hurricane lamps, bedding rolls, jars of strawberry jam, tins of biscuits and gumboots. Worst of all – I went blind! A burning red curtain for a few seconds then all was blackness. Fortunately I was still conscious and remembering the last image of the road ahead, I managed to keep the wheel steady while we slowed to a stop in a cloud of choking laterite dust.

"Gamal – I've gone blind", I said, quietly and dispairingly, dreading to put my worst fears into words. "I must have detached my retinas or severed my optic nerves in that crash. Everything went red then black and now I can't see a thing". For giving vent to rage or anger the

Arabic language must take some beating and Gamal now appeared to be exploring its profanity potential with some vehemence. To me his answer in English, when it came a few seconds later, was to the point and infinitely comforting.

"It's a box of red chilli pepper", he said, "It's everywhere. Hang on a second and I'll fetch some water to rinse your eyes". He brought the canvas water carrier from the front wing mirror (where it keeps the water delightfully cool by evaporation while driving) and started to pour cupfuls of cold clear water gently into each eye in turn. A wonderful moment this – as my sight gradually returned to normal. Still blinking and coughing we began to take stock of the damage. Firstly the vehicle – nothing wrong there and no bits hanging off or lying in the road; but inside was a different story – a chaotic mess – a total jumble of all our food, clothes, equipment – all liberally coated with fine red powder – chilli pepper! With handkerchiefs over our faces everything was unloaded into the road, well thumped, the vehicle brushed out and then repacked. An hour later we were again on our way, scanning the road surface ahead with even greater vigilance and, having learned our lesson, slowing down markedly near the tops of hills.

The Waza Game Reserve was well organized, clean and comfortable, with excellent cuisine (Vivre la France!) but not so large or possessing so rich a variety of wildlife as those in East Africa. Two large herds of the beautiful black sable antelopes (*Hippotragus niger*) like sturdy black horses with huge curved sharply pointed horns sweeping back over their bodies, were a definite bonus and the saddle-billed storks, hammerkops, bitterns and other bird-life were there in abundance and accessible. The journey back was reasonably uneventful and enlivened by seeing the villages perched, well away from the road, high up among the large rocks and boulders, with a network of interlacing footpaths linking them all to one another and down to the road. Siting them so high, presumably, was to avoid the clouds of dust raised by passing vehicles and also for safety since they were not easily accessible. The huts were most attractive with very high and pointed conical thatching and the walls covered with yellowish brown ochre with bright colourful patterns painted over them.

By late afternoon the last of our drinking water had run out and the vehicle too was beginning to steam. We wedged the bonnet partly open with a tree branch collected from the roadside vegetation and carried on driving slowly. In this oppressive heat we were all parched and dreaming of glistening bottles of ice cold lager. After a little while the rough scrubland began to give way to signs of approaching 'civilisation'; first some advertising hoardings, then a lone petrol station (unfortunately closed!) and soon there were trees lining the streets while the laterite had given way to tarmac. By this time the attractive mud huts with their conical thatched roofs had been replaced with the ubiquitous and unlovely corrugated iron roofs. A little later the more individual and sophisticated residences, with driveways and ornamental well-manicured lawns began to appear. We were back in town.

One such entrance caught our eye – two huge brick pillars each with a lamp on top, two huge wrought-iron gates – wide open and extending a tacit invitation to explore the broad sweeping shrub-lined driveway up to a large and impressive residence, many of the windows of which were decorously lit.

"How about calling in here to fill our water bottles" suggested Gamal beside me, "It probably has a good safe well with clean water".

"Good idea", I replied. "It's worth a try – let's go in and ask". With that I swung the Landrover in through the gates and up the drive, eventually parking beside some very fine automobiles, the elegance of which suggested that we might soon be in somewhat superior and doubtless very surprised company. We climbed out, shaking the dust from our clothes and, as we started to approach the house, a servant in a long white gown and red Muslim cap came to meet us. He smiled and, speaking in French, said "You are welcome – please follow me"

"We just wish to fill our water bottles" we replied, falling in behind him. He made no reply but kept walking towards the house – everything was clearly under control

On entering the house we were greeted by yet another servant, similarly clad but armed with a large tray bearing several crystal glasses of wine – some red: some white. With a muttered "Merci beaucoup" we downed the first glass to slake our parched throats and, since they were still proffered, promptly took another, to sip in less barbaric fashion.

The first reception servant now beckoned us to follow him, which we did – into an inner room where we were confronted by a sea of elegantly dressed ladies and gentlemen, all now looking interestedly at these strangely attired and much dishevelled newcomers. All were African – all beautifully clad in colourful robes and sandals and, until we arrived, doubtless all chatting amicably among themselves. This was clearly a very formal civic or diplomatic reception party into which we had accidentally blundered.

The host – a shortish man, beautifully attired with a regal manner and an engaging smile came forward to meet us, with his hand extended in greeting. In our fractured French we apologised for our intrusion, thanked him for the warmth of his welcome and hospitality, complimented him on the excellence of his wines and quickly explained our need to refill our water bottles. We added that we were part of an international malaria survey team on our way back to Nigeria and, apologising again for our inadvertent intrusion into his privacy, started to withdraw.

He smiled broadly and said (in perfect English), "Your arrival among us is as welcome as it is unexpected but please refresh yourselves and join us until we have supplied you with all that you need for your journey". Then, still smiling broadly, he turned to explain the situation to his guests, who nodded their understanding and smiled their salutations.

He then called his servants to attend to our needs, to refill our glasses and pass round the plates of typically French 'haute cuisine' – known more prosaically in Nigeria as 'small chop'!

When we finally took our leave of them, with many handshakes and their expressions of "Bon chance" and "Bon voyage" (but significantly no "au revoirs"!), the water carriers had been refilled, the Landrover radiator topped up and its windscreen and windows well washed. We thanked the waiting servants in the time-honoured fashion and, leaving them waving and grinning happily, drove off to look for the Customs Post, to cross back into Nigeria, before it closed for the night.

We learned the sad news of resistance on our return. The spraying campaign had been highly successful having reduced the overall malaria infection rate in the protected area almost to zero, while those living in the untreated control villages outside were almost 95% infected. But the failure of the DDT to kill adult mosquitoes couldn't be ignored and the W.H.O. Steering Committees in Geneva and in the Brazzaville African Regional Office decided that the project had to be scaled down and the well-trained Nigerian medical staff left to try to hold the new low-level of transmission. This was to be done by the regular administration and free issue of chloroquine syrup to all infants, schoolchildren, pregnant and nursing women and also made freely available on demand to all others.

But before finally leaving Nigeria we had two local ceremonies to enjoy; one the famous Argungu Fishing Festival – where the river is dammed for several weeks and filled with fish of all sizes. Some of the Nile Perch (Giwan Ruwa) weighed over 200 lbs and were 6 ft in length. Hundreds of fishermen were all squatting along the bank waiting for his Excellency the Sultan of Sokoto to say 'Go' and blow the whistle. Then it was literally a case of bottoms up and heads down under, to grope for the fish with hand and net. Catches were dragged out to the bank, weighed, recorded, killed and cut up for immediately sale to the crowds waiting to buy. The other momentous occasion was the Emir of Gwandu's ceremonial procession to celebrate Id el Fitr (Pl.17) – at the end of the fasting. This was extremely colourful with much music, drumming and dancing – the Emir and most of the dignitaries wearing exotic flowing robes (Rigas) delicately scented and bedecked with yards of tulle and coloured turbans. Most were mounted on gaily caparisoned horses in full regalia with attendants trotting along beside them carrying large colourful sun shades. This finished up with a Durbar in the local playing fields – where all kinds of competitive sports were offered – sword-swallowing, fire-raising. wrestling, one man vigorously chewing up small sharp nails and razor blades – apparently without harm – plenty of horsemanship displays and gymnastics – all giving rise to clouds of dust.

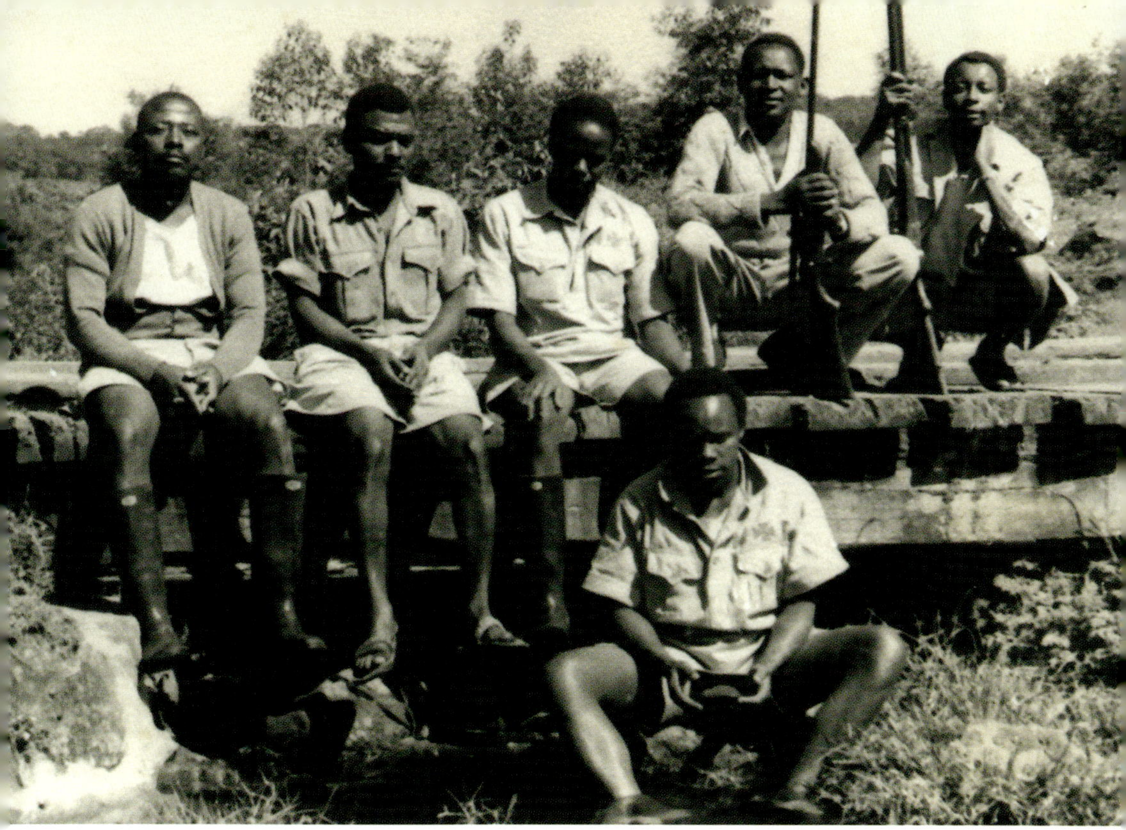

Above: *Plate 12.* IBD staff at Kerugoya – Trichinella studies in Southern Mt Kenya
Below left: *Plate 13.* Golbanti – journey up-river from Ngao to Golbanti, Kenya coast
Below right: *Plate 14.* Parasitology laboratory at Birnin Kebbi, N. Nigeria

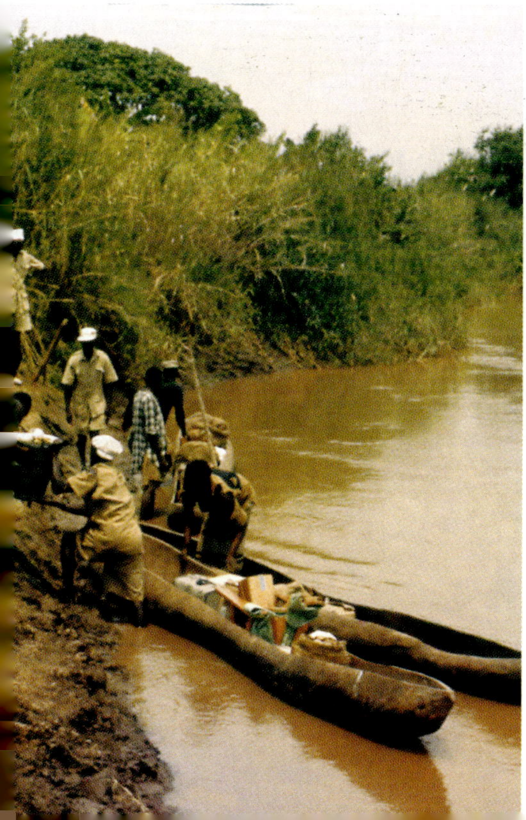

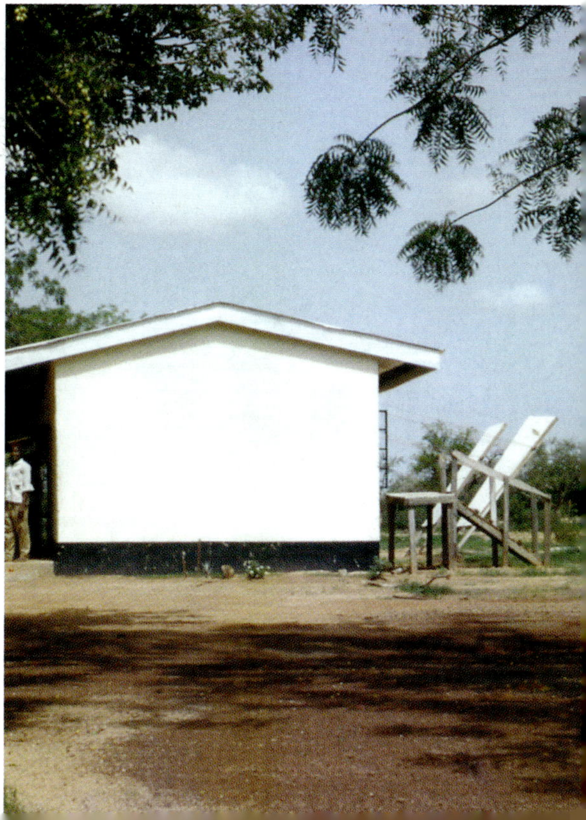

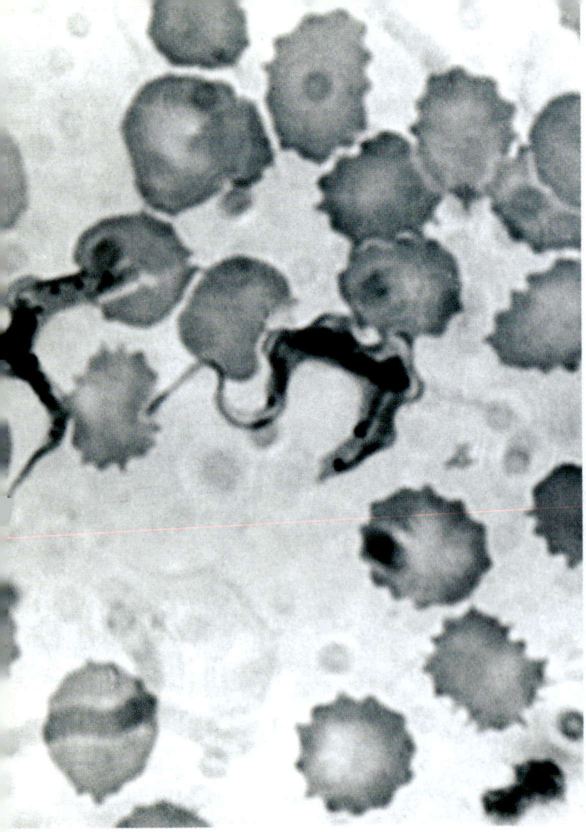

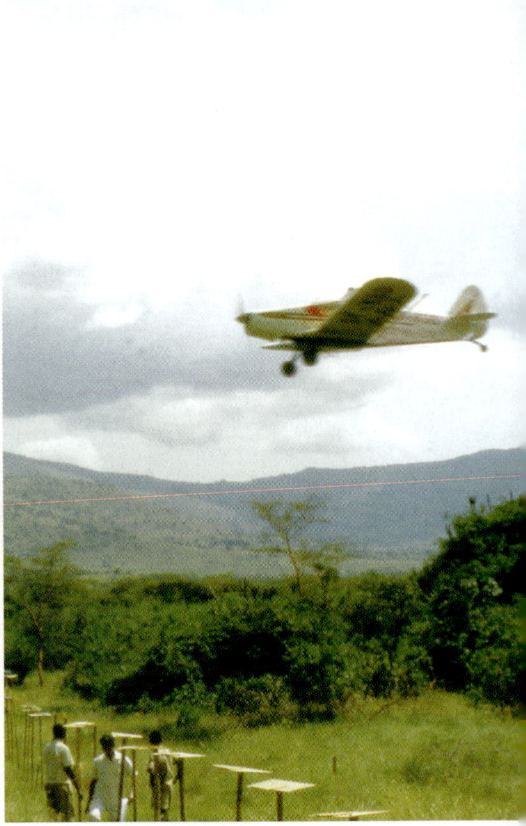

Above left: *Plate 15.* Sleeping sickness trypanosomes in thin blood-film (x400 magnification)

Above right: *Plate 16.* Airspray droplet analysis – flying over 'jump cards', Lambwe Valley

Below: *Plate 17.* Emir of Gwandu's parade at Birnin Kebbi, N. Nigeria

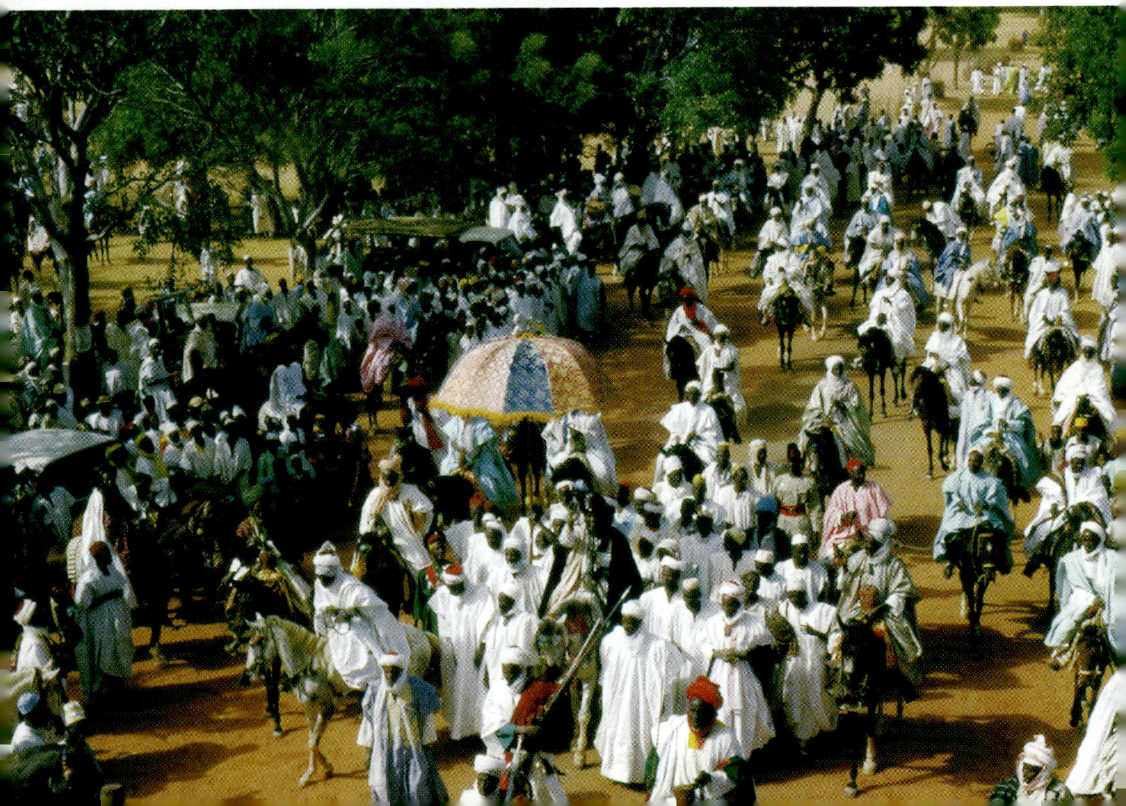

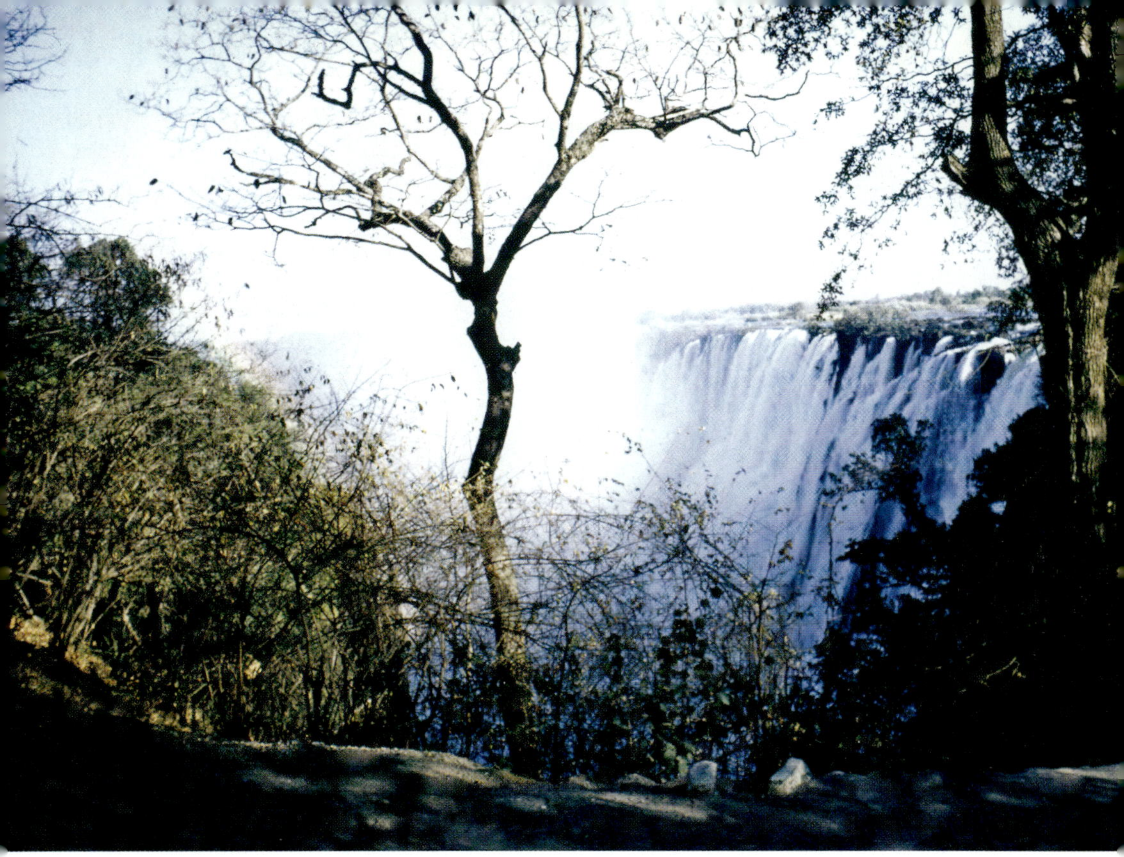

Above: *Plate 18.* Mosi-oa-tunya (Victoria Falls), Livingstone, Southern Province, Zambia
Below: *Plate 19.* Palpating swollen neck glands of sleeping sickness case, Zambia

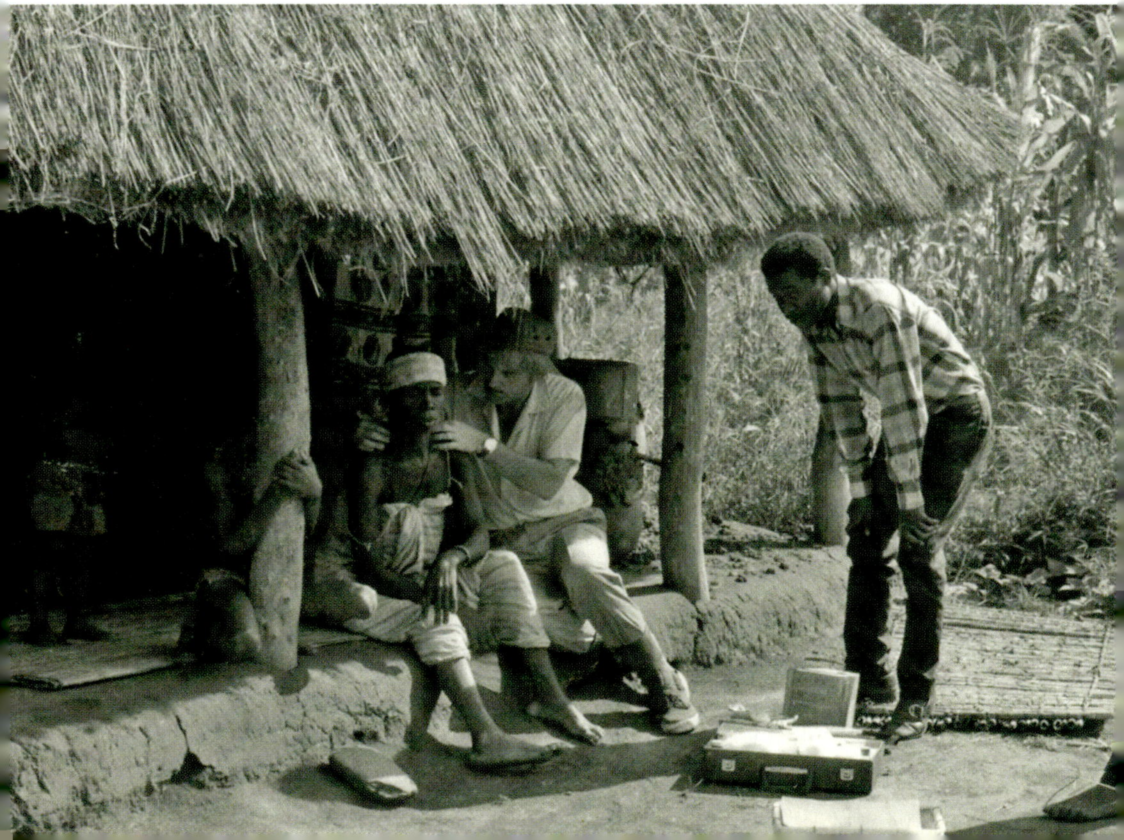

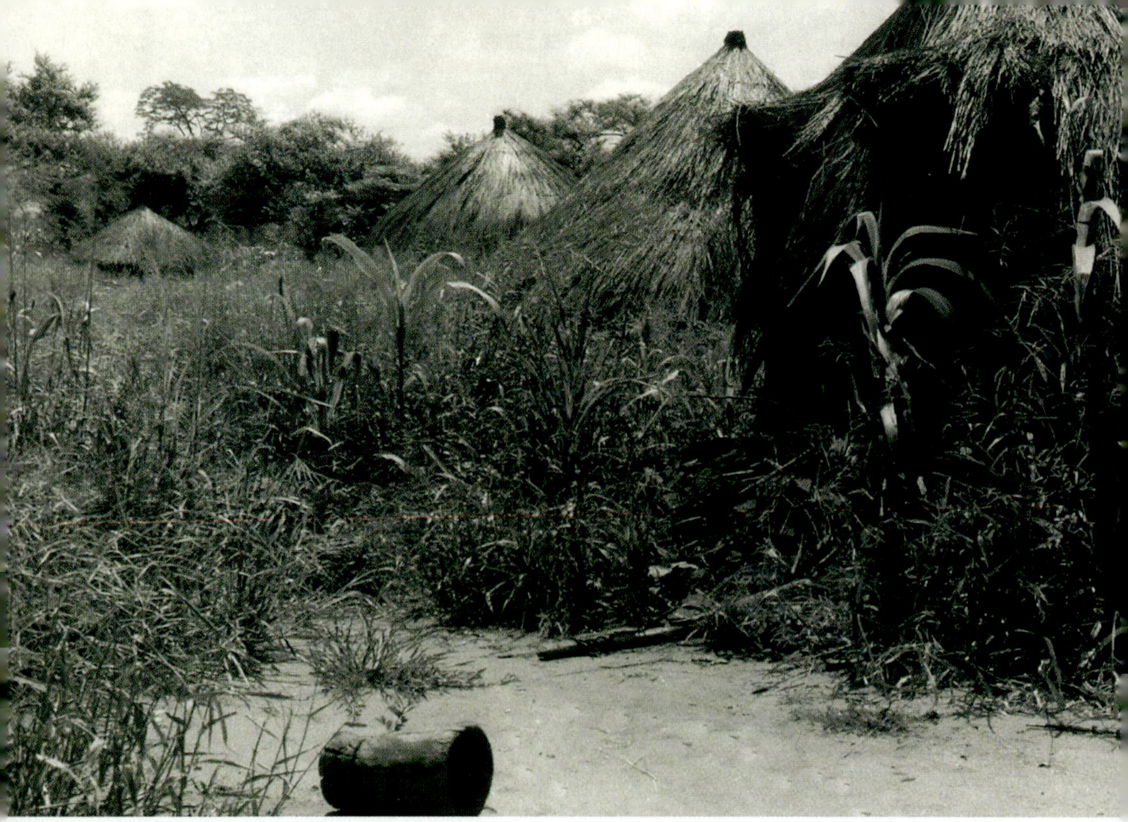

Above: *Plate 20.* Kanukawanga hamlet – deserted, tsetse-infested and reverting to bush, Zambia

Below: *Plate 21.* Chimanganya village – home of Yemi Daka – deserted and reverting to bush

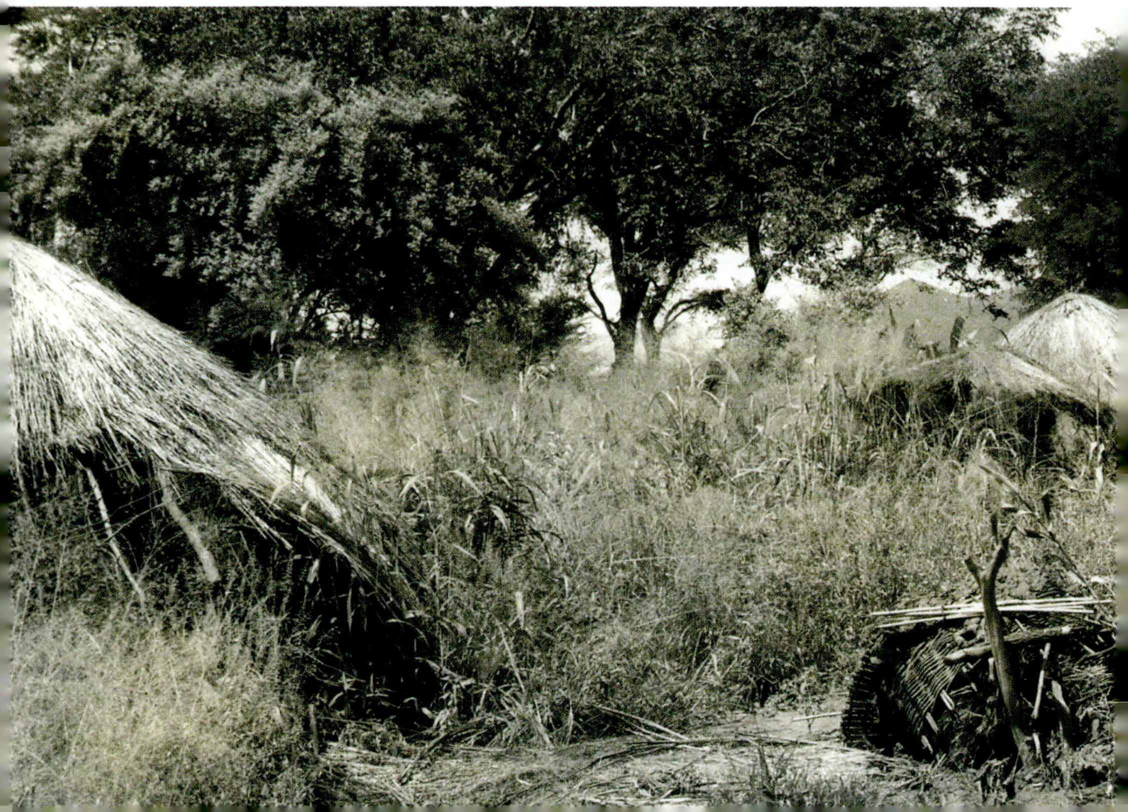

CHAPTER 13

Reassigned to Ghana

Working with the malaria unit in Ho, Volta Region – design new string-powered centrifuge (made by Prof. Alan Nunn May) to concentrate malaria parasites.

Due to the almost total lack of fresh fruit and vegetables combined with the oppressive heat and lack of electricity, my wife and I decided that it would be best if she took both children back to England; it was strangely quiet without them. But now, since the project was already being disbanded and I had been reassigned to work in Ghana, I decided to load all remaining possessions into the Peugeot Stationwagon and drive it firstly down to Lagos – then on along the coast through Cotonou (Benin), Lomé (Togo) to Aflao in southern Ghana before heading northwards to Ho in the Volta Region.

Passing through the duplicate sets of Immigration and Customs posts on both sides of each border took up an inordinate amount of time and tried one's patience to the full! Dressed in 'a little brief authority' some African officials can, if they so wish, makes one's life a misery – but a ready smile with a 'thank you' usually helps to oil the wheels of officialdom. Only when they are dressed in combat fatigues and armed with the ubiquitous AK47 (Kalashnikov) machine rifles are they many times more frighteningly unpredictable, especially if they have been drinking!. Despite heavy and continuous rain the car ran beautifully with no punctures or cracked springs – horribly overladen as she was and the road badly potholed and corrugated.

Gunter Kudicke, the W.H.O. malariologist in Ghana, was German – a cheerful bustling man and a very talented violinist and raconteur. His father had been a medical officer working with Drs. Koch and Taute in what was then Tanganyika, during the first world war. We found the Ghanaians extremely friendly and welcoming. The tennis club was a major social centre with plenty of tournaments and much social activity. For this latter the net was removed and the court immediately became a very busy dance floor with plenty of 'highlife' and old-fashioned waltzes – interspersed with equally active refreshment sessions with excellent cold 'Star' beers and large plates of yam chips. The local army officers club extended a permanent invitation to attend their cinema evenings which were always crowded and spiced with plenty of humorous comments from the audience!

At Ho the malaria unit was very efficiently run by Dr. Beausoleil with his team of scientists and technicians and really had no need for our additional expertise. When transport was available we were able to extend the malaria database by visits to outlying villages but this very hardworking and clearly very competent Ghanaian malariologist really had no need of us. Fortunately I was given permission to continue with my parasite concentration experiments aimed chiefly at detecting the low level infections that are particularly common in the older children and adults. This suppression of parasite levels is due to the build up of specific, natural acquired immunity resulting from constant reinfections from the bites of malaria-positive mosquitoes over the years. The unborn baby is given some degree of passive conferred immunity transplacentally and later receives more in the mother's milk but this is short-lived and disappears within the first few months after birth. If the child manages to survive until the age of 2-3 years, each new infection will add to a slowly growing body of natural immunity which, if not seriously impaired by malnutrition or other damaging infection, will serve to protect him or her against the worst ravages of malaria in later years.

The overthrow of President Kwame Nkrumah came whilst I was in Ho and was clearly greeted with much relief – with much spontaneous dancing in the streets and open-air parties. But later there were two further coups – both by the military – the second resulting in the death of a very popular soldier – Col. E.K. Kotaka. The mourning period lasted for several days and in Ho, as elsewhere, each of the local communities, led by their Chiefs, paraded through the streets of Ho in groups – periodically firing off loud volleys with their 'dane' shotguns with much noise and smoke making all the dogs bark! All were dressed alike with the colour of the village and all wearing the red headband of mourning. It was a very impressive and moving ceremony. The main airport in Accra was later named after him.

Because of the difficulties of finding malaria positives among the many blood-films being examined daily, in Birnin Kebbi (where every one had to be fully investigated) I began to explore means of examining larger volumes of blood, i.e. more than the finger prick samples taken routinely. Since the malaria parasites are only in the red blood cells, if these could be isolated from the liquid plasma and white cells etc, more could be examined per sample, thus increasing the sensitivity of the microscopic examination and giving a more accurate result. The simplest way to do this is to collect larger volumes of blood from the finger-prick into glass capillary tubes and spin these in a centrifuge. The solid heavier red cells would be packed in the lower part of the spun sample so that when the tube was etched and broken just above the top of the cells a film could be made from the contents. This showed very promising results and attracted the attention of those 'higher up'.

Now, in Ghana, with more time to spare for research, I started to investigate the possibility of differentially changing the specific gravity of the parasitised red cells so that, during subsequent centrifugation they would come more closely together in the packed cells. This was done by making up a range of saline solutions from almost pure water up to isotonic 8.2% normal physiological saline (that has no osmotic effect on human blood cells). From a bottle of malaria-infected human blood three capillary tubes were half filled with blood then topped up with the appropriate saline dilution. Having three for each sample would allow them to be cut high up, in the middle and low down after centrifugation – in order to locate where the parasitised cells had congregated (if at all!).

Later, when the samples had been spun and thin films made a strange phenomenon was noted. The banana-shaped malaria gametocytes (sexual forms) were found to be massively increased and drawn into the centre as the spreader moved across the slide when making the film. With a saline concentration of just over 7.0% this gave almost a X 40 concentration factor – a result as remarkable as it was unexpected!. When the slides were later examined by Professor Bruce-Chwatt, the senior malaria specialist in W.H.O./ H.Qs he compared the saline slide gametocyte count with that for the standard control thick blood films and found them to be twice as many. (when stained a normal thick blood film has a concentration factor of approximately X 20 over the relevant thin blood film).

Because of this encouraging result I was firstly rewarded by two scientific study visits – one to Professor Corredetti in Rome, a malariologist of international renown: the other to Professor Sir Ian MacGregor – an equally famous malariologist then heading the well known research centre at Fajara in the Gambia.. On my return I was asked to follow up my earlier studies using the infinitely more suitable facilities and the expert advice and guidance of the Director, with Dr. Mac Dowling (Malariologist) and Gerry Shute (Chief Technical

Scientist). at the W.H.O. Malaria Eradication Training School in Yaba, Lagos. This went well and resulted in our designing and field testing a new string-operated disc centrifuge based on the child's contra-rotating toy. This was not entirely original since a Professor Bo Holmstedt in the Karolinska Institute, Stockholm, had devised a slim banana-shaped device, also string operated, that had grooves to take 8 lengths of heparinised polyethylene tubing Although very fast it was considered not safe enough for field use since it had no cover to seal in the tubes. Our circular model held 20 capillary tube blood samples and packed the red cells in 4-5 minutes. When field tested for malaria diagnosis this showed a small but significant increase in positivity and was written up for publication in the W.H.O./MAL series.

Back in Ghana I ordered some new and better equipment from Geneva but sadly only a few days before it arrived I received a telex to say that I had been selected to join a new prestigious field epidemiological research team working on sleeping sickness in the Lambwe Valley, South Nyanza, Kenya, and which I was expected to join in a couple of weeks. This was a World Bank/U.N.D.P./W.H.O./ Kenya Government major programme – the first of its kind in Africa. I could now do no more than pack up all this equipment and drive with it down to the National Institute of Medical Research at the University of Ghana campus at Legon near Accra. I explained the situation to the Director (Dr. Saakwa-Mante) and to Professor Alan Nunn May- then holding the chair in solid state physics with whom I had been invited to work. He was a quiet and charming man, extremely helpful and full of good ideas – as well he might, being a nuclear physicist involved with the development of the atom bomb! He was now happily settled in Ghana after his earlier problems. Before my final departure from Ghana I decided to field-test the value of the sedimentation technique in a practical way. I selected one of the village schools, a few miles into the bush from Ho, one that we had not previously surveyed for malaria.

The headmaster was happy to participate as were the children when we explained what we were doing.. We took standard thick and thin blood-films from all children and, at the same time took capillary blood samples which the children watched us put through the range of saline solutions. We spun these on a 12v centrifuge linked to the vehicle battery and made a further batch of samples. The donation of a new football as a 'thank-you' present for the children brought a spontaneous roar of approval followed immediately by an explosive exodus to the fields outside – where the game (if such it could be called, with no whistles or referees to worry about and played in bare feet) was soon in full swing! Back in the malaria laboratory microscopy of the samples showed three times as many children positive for *P.falciparum* gametocytes in the saline-sedimented samples over the standard slides. This was a potentially valuable finding since it is only these gametes that are capable of initiating a new infection when taken up into the stomach of the vector mosquito.

One memorable Christmas was spent en famille at Elmina along the Cape coast. The white castle there had been notoriously active during the slaving days. The dungeons and underground tunnels through which the slaves were spirited out into waiting ships still seemed to echo the cries and protests of the luckless occupants. The treacherous sloping beach offshore with its hidden and dangerous undercurrents precluded swimming but the launchings and landings of the large and colourfully painted fishing canoes through the surf were carried out with great skill and much good humour. We were able to buy fresh fish straight from the boats.

On the morning of our departure from Ghana we had a disastrous breakfast (which included some fungus-infected wheat flakes) with some friends. My wife, not wishing to offend our host, ate the flakes and by the time we had reached the new Volta Dam settlement, en route to Accra airport, she became very sick and was admitted to the Volta Dam hospital. Believing that she was in good hands and would follow very shortly, and not being able to contact either Kenya or Geneva to warn them of my delay, I decided to go on ahead. This was a despicable thing to have done and I still feel thoroughly ashamed at not having stayed with her. Fortunately her illness was only temporary and she arrived in Kenya couple of days later.

CHAPTER 14

Sleeping Sickness Research in Kenya

A World Bank/W.H.O. – funded project in the
Lambwe Valley, Kenya

The project working area was the Lambwe Valley – a beautiful part of western Kenya (South Nyanza) where the Olambwe river runs down to the Victoria Nyanza (Lake Victoria) from the Kisii highlands, just south of the Kavirondo Gulf. Based first in temporary accommodation in Kisumu we commuted weekly into the work area. The road ran through colourful rolling country at first but, from Mirogi – a small village with a general Indian-run store – it became a red dirt road badly corrugated and a skating rink and a trap for the unwary in the rains!

The camp was situated along the crest of an escarpment that commanded a magnificent, almost aerial, view of the whole valley, sweeping away down to the valley floor, with the mountain masses on either side, out to the distant lake. Dr. Ken Willett, a medical doctor had worked for many years at the famous sleeping sickness research centres at Shinyanga and Tinde in north-western Tanzania; more recently he had been the Director of the West African Trypanosomiasis (difficult to say for some!) Research Centre in northern Nigeria. He was now chosen by W.H.O. to head the research team. Ken Willett had been a peace-time Flying Officer pilot in the RAF but had lost a leg in a plane crash and had turned to a career in medicine. He began by selecting team members with a known track record in Sleeping Sickness research. Since I had no previous experience with sleeping sickness, save that of being one of five volunteers to be given test inoculations by Dr. Heisch – though fortunately saved by the bell, as mentioned earlier, when Charlie Guggisberg, the first of Heisch's human 'guinea pig' volunteers, fell to the canvas (actually a concrete floor) with a temp of 104 and his peripheral blood swarming with highly motile trypanosomes, I was extremely surprised to be selected – but highly delighted to join such an illustrious group working on a subject that had first drawn me back to Africa. As it turned out it was my all-round laboratory and field experience and my lack of previous knowledge of sleeping sickness that did the trick. Dr. Willett had gambled that someone coming fresh to the subject would look at things with an unbiased eye and perhaps come up with new ideas. Given his usual lack of success with 'liar-dice' this could have been a disastrous choice!

The Kenya Government Project Co-Manager was Jan LeRoux who ran the Tsetse Control Department at the Kabete Veterinary laboratories near Nairobi ably aided by Bill Langridge (Tsetse Biologist) and Bert Shillinglaw – a small Scottish dynamo who arranged all the earlier field activities for large-scale tsetse control such as bush-clearing ('chain-dozing') and ground-spraying insecticide, mostly in the Roo Valley. Chain-dozing is a spectacular process and involves dragging a huge anchor chain weighing several tons between two large D8 tractors to uproot and clear bushes and small trees in which the tsetse rest.

The first general look at the valley was done from the air, in a plane hired from the Kenya Police Air Wing and expertly piloted by Senior Inspector 'Punch' Bearcroft – despite the fact of his having only one arm. Team members joked that when Ken Willett flew with him the fact that such flights normally cost 'an arm and a leg' was of no consequence and was thus reasonably priced! The Olambwe river flows down from the Kisii Highlands to Lake Victoria (Nyanza) – just south of the Kavirondo Gulf. The final approach to the valley, from Kisumu via Mirogi, was spectacular. Coming over the brow of the hill the ground falls away sharply leaving the eyes looking out into space – the enormous bulk of the lake lying in a haze some 10-12 miles away and below, almost at one's feet, the Lambwe valley laid out like a map with the river winding its way across the valley floor through the dense grey-green mass of the bush thicket and, behind it, the massive bulk of the Gwembe and Gwassi mountains, each with their steep thicket-filled gullies sweeping down to the valley floor at their feet. The project camp buildings were strung out along the edge of the escarpment at the head of the valley. Way down below were clusters of circular thatched huts and tiny figures with occasional wisps of smoke rising up from the woodfire and curling up in the still air. This feeling of space in such a vast amphitheatre was heightened by the faint but crystal clear small sounds and voices coming up from below and also by the huge flocks of black and white Abdim storks spiralling lazily and drifting slowly across the valley – 'aloft, incumbent on the lonely air'. Behind the Gwembe and Gwassi mountains is the Mara river with its justly famed Game reserve, and the Serengeti Plains stretching down to the Ngorongoro Crater and to Mwanza, the major port at the south end of Lake Victoria, seen by the explorer Speke and which led him eventually to discover the source of the Nile. The nearby Speke Gulf was named after him.

The Lambwe Valley itself is some 3-4 miles wide and covered for the most part by the impenetrable 'Ruma' lantana thicket which supported an enormous population of *Glossina pallidipes* tsetse-flies – feeding almost exclusively on the many species of wild animals, but always more than willing to top up with some tasty fresh human blood! Patches of more open vegetation away from the river proper housed fair numbers of *Glossina morsitans* the open woodland tsetse – also feeding on game but even more willing to take blood feeds from humans. Direct crossing of the valley was impossible except for a single path cut through the thicket. But the soil was the notorious 'black cotton' which became glutinous and a tenacious enemy of all motor vehicles in the rainy season. The road also allowed easier access to the many small-holdings that were springing up both outside and, such was the land hunger, eventually also inside the protective fence of the Game Reserve; and this despite the attentions of the Game Ranger and his staff based in a small camp up on the escarpment just below the W.H.O. Research Station.

These African settlers were living off subsistence crops of maize and millet with protein supplementation from the illicit poaching of the wild animals, a fact that was soon reflected in an increasing number of Sleeping Sickness cases. These animals are the natural hosts of the parasites (trypanosomes) and are often present in the tsetse flies feeding on them and transmitting the infections. 'Game animals' were generally abundant in most parts of the Valley and even came up close to the camp built along the escarpment. These included the reedbuck (with their characteristic whistle which we often heard in the evenings), oribi, bushbuck, Jacksons hartebeest, kudu, waterbuck, buffalo, giraffe, sable antelope, duikers, the beautiful nocturnal bat-eared foxes, serval cats, leopards and cheetah but, alas, no lions, elephants or rhinos.

Until the comparatively recent advent and spread of the HIV/AIDS retro-virus and the global spread of drug-resistant strains of malaria, of all the tropical diseases that beset sub-Saharan Africans, perhaps the most dramatic are the trypanosomiases – causing sleeping sickness in humans and the wasting and lethal disease 'Nagana' in their domestic livestock. The fact that some 4.5 million square miles of African woodland are almost totally devoid of domestic animals and human habitation, due to the presence of the vector tsetse-fly, bears tacit witness to the lethality of this disease for man and beast alike; while the sleeping sickness epidemic that raged around the shores of Lake Victoria during the first few years of the last century, killing well over 200,000 villagers, is a constant and sobering reminder of the degree of devastation that this disease can cause in a unprotected population that seems to have no natural immunity to this disease.

The association of this invariably fatal (if untreated) human disease with the drooling, shuffling, emaciated and mentally confused sufferer, gives rise to the mystique that often attaches to sleeping sickness in the minds of many villagers, for whom these symptoms, understandably, have sinister and dire connotations. To the medical or veterinary scientist the complexities of sleeping sickness epidemiology and epizootiology pose a challenging array of problems; to an immunologist, charged with the task of developing effective vaccines against these parasites, the phenomenon of 'antigenic variation' (the constant changing the nature of the outer infective coat of the trypansomes) presents a formidable obstacle, while the organisms themselves have intrigued, delighted and frustrated investigators from the turn of the 20th Century until the present day. They have attracted many devoted and careful studies but their behaviour remains uncomfortably unpredictable'.

In sub-Saharan Africa this disease is perpetuated within a complex ecosystem, one involving the parasites (trypanosomes), the vector tsetse-flies, certain game animal reservoir hosts on which they normally feed and man and his domestic livestock. However, only a small proportion of these parasites circulating in nature are infective for man and for long they defied all attempts by the early researchers to produce a diagnostic technique which identified those infective for man – save for inoculation of the suspect organisms into human volunteers. Understandably these were few and far between! Nevertheless, several of the early scientists bravely inoculated such strains into themselves, such was their dedication to the cause!

Because of this difficulty the nature and extent of the mammalian reservoir could not be identified with certainty (nor is it fully understood today, despite significant progress in diagnostic methods – see later); indeed the consensus of opinion has for long considered that the numbers presently diagnosed represent only the very small tip of a very large iceberg. The latest pandemic to sweep across Africa from west to east in 1999–2001, from Mali to Ethiopia and down to Angola and Mozambique, produced more than 600,000 new clinical cases with more than 50,000 deaths.

Another serious economic factor of the trypanosomiases is the continuing exclusion of livestock from some 10 million square kilometres of tsetse-infested land that would otherwise be suitable for cattle ranching or diary farming, providing valuable meat, milk hides and skins and oxen for ploughing. Much earlier, during his missionary travels in southern Africa, Dr. David Livingstone had drawn attention to the disastrous effects of this disease when he lost 43 of his cattle and was unable to find the cause.

The more chronic form of this disease (*Trypanosoma brucei gambiense*) was known in West Africa more than 600 years ago and records show that the slave traders in those days were well aware of the fatal 'negro lethargy', which they recognised by the swollen posterior cervical lymph glands at the base of the neck known as 'Winterbottom's sign' – named after the British physician who in 1803 described this fatal lethargy and its symptoms. The method by which these swollen glands were often excised, in a futile attempt to arrest the course of the infection, and described in lurid and harrowing detail by the traveller Roger Casement, would seem to the modern reader almost as lethal as the disease itself! The more acute form (*Trypanosoma brucei rhodesiense*) was first discovered in the Luangwa Valley, Zambia, in south-eastern Africa, from which it is believed to have spread steadily northwards through Tanzania, Kenya and Uganda to Ethiopia, where it appeared for the first time, in epidemic form, in 1967.

Tsetse-borne trypanosomes were first discovered by Bruce in 1895, and named after him, whilst he was working with his wife on the closely-associated cattle disease 'nagana' in northern Zululand; but they were not known to infect man until the turn of the century when, in 1901, a surgeon named Fords first saw them in the blood of a febrile British captain of a steamboat plying on the river Gambia in West Africa. The highly motile organisms were described and named (*T.b.gambiense*) but were not at the time recognised as the causal agents of the well-know West African sleeping sickness or 'negro lethargy' but only of the relatively mild 'trypanosomal fever'. The establishment of the Congo Free State in 1885 and the exploration and development of trade along the riverine travel routes that followed, permitted soldiers and labourers employed in the upper reaches of the Congo River and its tributaries to carry the sleeping sickness infections, acquired in the endemic coastal regions, thus spreading the disease into new areas. By 1905 a vast region, stretching from the Lulua tributary eastwards for 250 miles to the shores of Lake Tanganyika, had been invaded. It has been estimated that between 1896 and 1905 about half a million people died of sleeping sickness in the Congo Basin.

At the same time another epidemic began in the Busoga District of Uganda, some hundres of miles further east on the norther shores of Lake Victoria (Nyanza). Although discontinuous with the epidemic area of the Congo, the Busoga outbreak was attributed to infections carried by the disaffected soldiers and followers of Emin Pasha when they were brought down by Lugard between 1892-5 from Emin's old headquarters on the Albert Nile. These had been infected presumably from members of Stanley's Emin Pasha Relief Expedition when stationed in the area to the south of Lake Albert. Within five years of its start in South Busoga in 1901, this *T.b.gambiense* epidemic had decimated the populations living along the shores and on the islands of Lake Victoria. The total mortality due to sleeping sickness alone in Uganda, up to the end of 1906 considerably exceeded 200,000.

This epidemic was finally brought under control when the Governor, Sir Hesketh Bell, acting on his own initiative, persuaded the Chiefs to move their people and the villages inland to higher ground, some two miles away from the tsetse-fly infested lakeside regions, thus breaking the close man-tsetse contact. By then the extent of the devastation was appalling; some of the Sesse islands had lost every soul, while in others a few moribund natives were crawling about in the last stages of the disease – all that were left of a once-teeming population. Christy, a visiting doctor, contributed another 'vignette', which must have been sadly typical of the time...'At a small hamlet in Buvuma I saw three little children playing outside a hut in which the father was lying in the last stages of sleeping sickness; in an adjacent hut lay a woman also in the late stage of the infection with terrible ulcers on her thighs and ankles; while in a field close by was a youth, also seriously ill, unable to stand, crying and talking hysterically, as he endeavoured to scoop a hole in the sun-baked ground in the hope of finding one last remaining sweet potato in a patch long out of cultivation'.

This outbreak prompted the British Government to set up a three-man commission to study the cause of sleeping sickness and its mode of transmission. The team, consisting of Drs. Low, Christy and Castellani, left for Uganda in 1902. The Rev. Dr. Wiggins, himself well used to the vagaries of life in East African, having been posted from the comforts of Mombasa to the uncertainties of Kisumu on the strength of a hoax telegram, when he met the party in Kisumu, thought them a 'queer lot'; in fact disagreements between Low and Christy over the leadership of the party and the labelling of their reserved railway carriage, had reportedly led to fisticuffs on the platform at Mombasa station! Although they eventually reached

Uganda safely they were unable to identify the causal agent and soon Christy and Low returned to Britain, but Castellani stayed on to follow up his belief in a streptococcal (bacterial) causation. But although he also noted (and recorded) the presence of the highly motile trypanosomes in the cerebro-spinal fluid of several sleeping sickness cases, he failed to confirm its significance. This was left to Drs Bruce and Nabarro, who had joined Castellani in 1903 as members of the second sleeping sickness commission and who later shared, with him, the credit for discovering the cause of this disease. The tsetse-fly (*Glossina palpalis*) was also incriminated by Bruce and his colleagues as the vector – although other species were later identified as additional vectors.

At this time the epidemiological situation seemed to be fairly clear; there was one trypanosome (*Trypanosoma brucei gambiense*) capable of infecting man – while others, incuding *Trypanosoma brucei brucei* infected game and domestic animals. However, in 1910 an event occurred which was to give rise to more speculation, debate and bitter controversy than almost any other aspect of this disease. In 1908 two mineral prospectors from what is now Zimbabwe, were badly bitten by tsetse while travelling in the Luangwa Valley, in Northern Rhodesia (now Zambia). While they would have come into contact with other species of tsetse flies (*Glossina morsitans*, *G.pallidipes* and *G.brevipalpis*) it is certain that they never passed through country infested with *G.palpalis*. In a little over 6 months both men had succumbed to trypanosome infections that were clearly much more virulent than any seen previously. These were later named *Trypanosoma brucei rhodesiense*.

Immediately and almost inevitably a controversy arose over the relationship between *T.b.rhodesiense* and *T.b.brucei*. One school of thought, typically represented by the Germans Taute (1913), Kleine (1914) and Taute & Hüber (1919) maintained that the two organisms were separate and distinct species. Others, notably Kinghorn & Yorke (both keen Liverpool supporters!) believed them to be identical. Working at this time in the Luangwa Valley, Kinghorn & Yorke (1914) found the 16% of all the game animals they examined had, in their blood, trypanosomes indistinguishable from the *T.b.rhodesiense* found in human cases.

On this evidence, that the wild game animals constituted the main reservoir from which the tsetse flies (*Glossina morsitans* in particular) derived trypanosomes that were pathogenic to man and to his domestic livestock, Bruce and his colleagues held that, because of the morphological and physiological similarities of the all the trypansome samples collected (findings which have since been confirmed many times), the trypanosomes found in human sleeping sickness cases and in the wild game animals were identical and that all trypanosomes found in animals could infect man.

However, this view was held to be untenable when it was realised that in some areas of sub-Saharan Africa these trypanosomes were present in animals but they were never found in man, despite his contact with tsetse flies in these areas. Bruce believed that, if the two organisms (*T.brucei* and *T.rhodesiense*) were truly identical, the distribution of sleeping sickness cases would coincide with that for *G.morsitans* and *T.brucei*. (the writer holds the view that *T.rhodesiense* evolves from *T.brucei* in animals when tsetse feeding on them start to feed on man). The presence of human blood elements in the tsetse fly gut inhibit the further multiplication of the 'brucei' elements (which are sensitive to human serum) and stimulate the change to the human-infective '*rhodesiense*' form.

With laudable Germanic persistence Taute (1913) was so convinced that these were different organisms that, having first selected an area apparently free from sleeping sickness, he very heroically inoculated himself with animal blood containing thousands of polymorphic trypanosomes (i.e. able to adopt many different shapes – a feature not shown by other trypanosomes – which do not infect man) and allowed himself to be bitten by infected tsetse flies. That he did not become infected was fortunate indeed, since there was, at that time, no known cure for sleeping sickness and an infection would quickly have been fatal. Later, while making a strategic retreat from the pursuing British armed forced in southern Tanganyika, Taute & Hüber (1919) found time to inoculate themselves and 129 other men with six different strains of polymorphic trypanosomes taken from naturally infected horses and mules – but no-one became infected.

This was very impressive evidence, yet it failed to convince the 'opposition', some of whom held that, although it had not been experimentally demonstrated that man could be infected with polrmorphic trypanosomes from game. It had been shown quite clearly that both game and domestic animals could be infected with trypanosomes taken from human cases. Thus, they argued, since tsetse were readily infected from these animals, it was difficult to understand how the parasites of man could fail to be widely disseminated amongst the game animals.

For the past sixty years or more one of the great obstacles to the study of the epidemiology and epizootiology of African trypanosomiasis has been this difficulty of distinguishing the non-human-infective *T.brucei* from the highly human-infective *T.rhodesiense*. For many years the only means available for making this distinction has been a direct test of infectivity in a human volunteer. This became possible with the discovery of the curative drug Suramin, for this disease, but for obvious ethical and practical reasons, such experimental identification could only very rarely be performed. Thus the nature and extent of the natural animal and insect reservoirs of sleeping sickness could not be established.

Evidence suggests that sleeping sickness has an element of periodicity, sudden outbreaks and epidemics appearing, usually in old and often long-quiescent foci, for reasons that are not understood. The most recent Sleeping Sickness pandemic in Africa at the turn of the last century (1999-2001) was certainly one such; but its rapid, disastrous and uncontrollable spread was almost certainly facilitated by the almost total lack of medical surveillance in the known danger areas. Had the villagers been checked regularly this would have given timely warning of an abnormal build-up of cases in the bush villages and alerted the medical and tsetse control services in good time. Like a forest fire – once well alight there is little that can be done to stop it, until it has run its course and died of its own accord, leaving the dead and abandoned villages as tacit evidence of the disaster.

Very early in the project Dr. Ken Willett, was moved to head the W.H.O./H.Qs sleeping sickness unit in Geneva. He had been running this new research programme, largely by radio and from his office close to his Government counterpart in Nairobi. His replacement was a Dr. David Scott a specialist sleeping sickness epidemiologist with many years experience in Ghana and Botswana. His first major decision was to move the project, lock-stock & barrel, out of Kisumu and into the Lambwe Valley – thus eliminating at a stroke the time-wasting and laborious business of commuting daily some 180 miles. Aided by local masons and carpenters individual houses, laboratories and toilet blocks were quickly put up and a large diesel generator installed for power and lighting. Working collectively we also built a large screened dining room with a bar, a fine verandah overlooking the valley, a kitchen block and a large library and reading room. Long-range radio communications were established with Nairobi and all teams working in the valley were equipped with walkie-talkies; these came in useful when vehicles were stuck in the black cotton soil or had broken down. Perched as it was along the top of the escarpment the camp was a veritable 'Shangri La' and at night, from the valley, looked a picture of fairy-lights.

This new team consisted of doctors and scientists (both medical and veterinary), entomologists, immunologists and veterinarians; these were joined by similar staff members of the Kenya Veterinary

& Tsetse Control Laboratories in Nairobi. The project had five objectives:-

1. To examine all the people and treat all who were infected (with Sleeping Sickness and any other diseases), try to establish where and when they became infected and which wild animals were acting as reservoirs for this disease.

2. To study the biting habits of the vector tsetse flies.

3. To study and try to improve methods of diagnosis – especially trying to identify human infective trypanosomes in the non-human hosts.

4. To evaluate different methods of killing the tsetse and eliminating/reducing Sleeping Sickness transmission.

A separate entomological research station was established on the lakeshore at Sindo, where the Roo Valley, an offshoot from the lower part of the Lambwe, ran out into the lake. This valley too was full of tsetse and was thus ideal for independent studies which could be carried out in comparative seclusion – away from the disturbing effects of the medical, veterinary and wildlife teams. The Game Ecologist (seconded from the FAO/Rome) located, identified, counted and examined most of the wild animals present. The Sindo-based entomologists, too, were studying tsetse numbers, identity and behaviour but, even more importantly, they also planned, directed and evaluated the effect of spraying the whole of the valley thickets with a powerful long-lasting (Dieldrex) insecticide – firstly from a helicopter and later with a small fixed-wing aeroplane. The latter operated from a landing strip in the valley just below the camp and on arrival from Nairobi, the pilot would first buzz the camp to ask for a vehicle to be sent down to collect the pilot and any passengers.

Although the helicopter was kept overnight at the project's helipad, during the spraying activities it was able to utilise any open space near to the thicket which the Landrovers could reach easily. This made for speedier turn-rounds when refilling with fuel or insecticide; another important benefit was the downwash of air from the propellor blades which swirled the insecticide droplets down through the canopy and on to the under sides of the leaves – a favourite site for resting tsetse flies. This fact had been established by the very relevant independent investigation and detailed study of tsetse behaviour, in a specially secluded part of the valley, by Dr. Donald Minter, the entomologist from the London School of Hygiene & Tropical. Medicine with whom I had earlier set out to catch the Langata leopard. His ingenuity and practical skills were put to particularly good use in the construction of a huge field study 'cage' which he built in part of the Ruma thicket. With its two-storey working platforms Donald was able to catch tsetse flies, mark them on the thorax with a small dab of irridescent paint and release them again. When subsequent scanned at night with an ultra-violet lamp the paint spots glowed up brightly providing valuable information about the resting locations inside the thicket -mostly on the undersides of the Lantana branches and leaves.

Medical officer Dr. Hubert Watson and I worked with the medical auxiliary staff seconded from the Division of Insect-Borne Diseases, Kenya Medical Department (my old 'alma mater'). Very ably assisted by their quiet, gentle and very experienced leader Joel Sawe, we examined and took blood samples from people of all ages living in the new illegal settlements (inside the protected game reserve!) and in nearby villages and hamlets – even those living in the small individual hamlets clinging to the sides of the Gwassi and Gwembe mountains (Pl.8). All positives for sleeping sickness or other serious conditions were brought up to the camp, appropriate samples (blood, CSF, urine etc) were taken for examination and the patients either treated or, if more seriously ill, taken immediately to the nearest hospital at Homa Bay. Here a special ward had been prepared and extra staff taken on to look after them. We used to visit them quite frequently to check their recovery and to obtain valuable epidemiological data on where they were likely to have been infected and their occupations (other than illicit game poaching and spirit distillation which were largely, and with reason, taken for granted!).

CHAPTER 15

A 'Tryp' or Two in Tsetse Country

Air-spraying tsetse flies – 'rugger tackling' antelopes at night – Gaudeusia (back from the dead) – characterising trypanosomes found in tsetse flies, game and domestic livestock

One effect of sleeping sickness infection is to diminish libido and one old patient whom we had earlier put into the Homa Bay hospital, when I visited him complained bitterly that he had lost his main interest in life i.e. that his prime member persistently refused to 'stand to attention' when required. I promised him ' a stand like an elephant' if he would only complete the full course of treatment. This brought a smile to his face and immediate compliance! Refusal to complete treatment was an on-going problem and invited drug-resistance and making the inevitable recurrence of the partially treated infections even more difficult to cure.

Reg the Game Ecologist, a strong, well-built young man and a keen rugby player, was responsible for identifying and counting the different wild animal species in the valley. For this he had to cut several transect lines through the thicket, a formidable task, and drive along them by day and also by night, since some animal species are active only after dark. We also had to collect blood samples from them to help identify which were acting as reservoir hosts for this disease. Because at that time dart-anaesthetising was both difficult and expensive, an easier method was to work at night dazzling each animal with the vehicle's spot-light, throwing a large capture net over it from close quarters and then taking the venous blood sample (usually from a neck or leg vein) whilst the helpers were holding it down. Many animals seemed mesmerised by the light and some would even advance along the beam almost up to the Landrover. However, since net-throwing was difficult to do in the dark, even with the spotlight, Reg decided to try rugger-tackling them – holding them still while others took the blood samples; at least that was the plan! The first (and last) attempt he made was on a fairly large reedbuck. We held the spotlight steady;

the animal, temporarily dazed, stood quite still and Reg took a short run and flung himself horizontally at it – aiming to embrace all four legs if possible. There was a very brief period of turmoil, a large cloud of dust was kicked up which momentarily masked the rapid disappearance from the scene of a very frightened (or affronted) reedbuck; when the dust cleared Reg could be seen trying to get up again, clutching the remnants of his shirt and trying to staunch the blood flowing freely from several wounds inflicted by four clearly very sharp hooves. Thereafter we used the anaesthetising dart-gun and retained the thrown net as a back-up.

When the rains came the medical team was in the middle of surveying hamlets along the lakeshore at the bottom of the valley To save the often quite difficult drives to and from the camp down the narrow, bumpy and now very slippery tracks, we decided to build a small subsidiary base at a strip of land jutting out into the lake known as Mbita Point. We put up tents for sleeping and erected two small metal 'bolt-together-panels' rondavels (one an office and the other a small laboratory) with a plinth for a small electric generator. It was an idyllic, pleasant and peaceful spot but, as we found out the first night, also a local hippodrome! The snortings and grunts as they came ashore to socialise and occasionally try to sort out their differences, left us all sadly bereft of sleep and much frightened as they stumbled into the tent guy ropes. By good fortune the hippos too, probably put off by our combined snorings, opted for privacy and thereafter came ashore further down the promontory and left us in peace. This lovely spot right on the lake shore later became a permanent medical research field station for the University of Nairobi. It's access to the lower end of the valley considerably shortened our driving and, being in direct line with the main camp, we started calling them in morse with a hand held lamp, whenever we wanted to talk to them on the radio.

Weekends were sometimes spent in Kisumu, first collecting our cars from the store in Mirogo run by the kindly Mehta family. Hubert and I joined the Kisumu Yacht Club, bought an old GP 14 sailing dinghy and started racing. Although named 'Pelorus Jack', after the famous dolphin that used to lead the sailing vessels into harbour at Auckland, New Zealand, sadly it displayed little of its name-sake's speed but instead gave us a good forward view of the Kisumu racing fleet in action!.

One very dangerous encounter with a poisonous snake occurred one late morning in the Lambwe Valley. I had just finished writing my report and the fact that I was moving quite fast out of the door (I had just been called for lunch!) probably saved my life. Lying immediately outside and sunning itself was a huge black mamba; it was thick as my leg and stretched the full length of the concrete plinth – about 15 feet. In my haste I could do nothing but jump clean over it and run quickly into the verandah, slamming the door behind me.

The black mamba is both aggressive and moves very fast over the ground; now disturbed by the shouts and vibrations it moved quickly into top gear with its head up high and swaying from side to side took off down the valley at great speed, probably hurling reptilian abuse and scornful jibes at the inaccuracy of those who, having arrived earlier for lunch, were now busy throwing stones at it.

One other snake occasion was really more humorous than dangerous. Hubert Watson, Joel Sawe and I were walking quickly in Indian file down a narrow path, having completed the mapping and examination of a small hamlet on the lower slopes of Gwembe mountain. I was leading and, as we still had a mile or so to reach camp in time for afternoon tea, we were swinging along fairly fast. Suddenly, a yard or so in front of me I saw two snakes, loosely coiled round each other in a writhing kind of dance. Their heads were about waist-high. I managed to put on all brakes and stopped suddenly; Hubert behind me had no visual warning and started climbing up my back while Joel, similarly unwarned, climbed up his. We finished up collapsing sideways into the grass laughing – in all probability the two snakes did likewise as they, too, went off home.

It was during the air-spraying programme that we had a strange plane buzz us before it flew off down to the landing strip in the valley below the camp. On board were veterinary/tsetse control scientists from Zambia bringing with them a 3-man Swedish camera team from a major Stockholm newspaper. Having spent a couple of days with us discussing techniques and filming all associated activities they took off to film some close-ups of the wild animals in the valley before heading back to Lusaka. Unfortunately in trying to get some really low shots, while flying slowly, probably due to the extra weight in the back and the drag from the open window the plane stalled and spun in; it was badly damaged but no-one was seriously injured. A radio-message to Lusaka called up another plane a day later to take them back. We later heard that the filming had been very successful and had created much interest back in Sweden.

Reg with his game scouts were coming back to camp late one evening when they saw a large elderly reedbuck lying sick beside the track. They lifted it into the Landrover and brought it up to us at the camp in the hopes of saving it. While John Robson the FAO vet was preparing what he hoped would be a life-saving injection, I took some blood from it looking for trypanosomes; and, sure enough, these it had in plenty. We quickly identified them as *T.b.brucei* group with a slight chance of their being the human-infective sleeping sickness 'rhodesiense' parasites. Despite John's best efforts the old reedbuck died shortly afterwards. Some of the blood had been frozen for later studies. But it had one further pleasant surprise for us for. While scanning the still wet blood under the microscope, stage by stage, I came across something that most trypanosomologists see only in textbooks – a megatrypanosome. This was huge – about a 100 microns in lengths and beautifully curvaceous! Its large undulating membrane was moving rhythmically and, to study it in more detail, I touched a small drop of alcohol under the coverslip. This slowed it down considerably and most of the camp members crowded round and were able to have a good look at it and compare it with the drawings in the text-books. We identified it as *Trypanosoma* (*Megatrypanum*) *ingens* from the drawing in Cecil Hoare's classical textbook '*The Trypanosomes of Mammals*'.

A few days later a report came in of a possible sleeping sickness case, from a small hamlet along the northern side of the valley, quite close to where the dying reedbuck had been found. The team investigates immediately and brought in a young woman named Gaudensia who, like the reedbuck, seemed all but dead. She had very shallow breathing, totally inert, her eyes had turned up. Immediate microscopical examination of the wet blood films showed many active trypanosomes 'kicking' about between the blood-cells (unlike malaria parasites trypansomes live outside the red cells). After a quick but thorough medical examination and a lumbar puncture (by David Scott), which also showed trypanosomes, Gaudensia was taken to the Homa Bay hospital and intravenous treatment with Mel B started. At that time Mel B (i.e. Melarsoprol) was the only drug that was effective against late-stage sleeping sickness infections – when the parasites had penetrated the blood-brain barrier and entered the cerebro-spinal fluid. It is the adverse effect of the parasites toxins on the surface of the brain that cause the severe symptoms – tremors, sudden sleeping, inability to walk, drowsiness and death. With *T.b.rhodesiense* this occurs about four to five weeks after infection of the blood and lymphatics. This is why it is so important to find cases early, by regular monthly surveillance of those living in known Sleeping Sleeping foci or who have recently come to live in close contact with tsetse flies; since it is only from these early infections of the blood and lymphatics that the tsetse become infected and pass on the parasites to every person it feeds on thereafter. The blood infection is very much easier to treat, with virtually a 100% certainty of a complete cure. We all thought that

Guadensia had little real chance of survival but she soon improved and made a complete recovery. We were all delighted, some time later, when she re-visited us at the camp with her husband and their new-born daughter.

By now the field surveys and mapping had been completed and David Scott asked me to concentrate on characterising all of the trypansome samples that had been collected from people, from wild and domestic animals and from dissected wild-caught tsetse fly salivary glands. This was in the hope of finding some means of differentiating the human-infective '*rhodesiense*' forms from the identical and far more prevalent non-human-infective '*brucei*'. Many of these 'unknowns' had been collected from naturally infected game animals, domestic livestock and from tsetse flies; they were still deeply frozen in liquid nitrogen cylinders. In the past some of these had failed to infect the human volunteers in which they had been tested and were proven 'bruceis'. For obvious reasons only very few of these existed and these were kept permanently in the cryobank as valuable reference material.

CHAPTER 16

A Valuable Discovery

Serendipitous discovery of a simple test for differentiating trypanosomes infective for man from those that are not (the B.I.I.T.) – a commendation from U.N. and W.H.O.

The inability to differentiate *T.b.rhodesiense* (capable of killing man in a few short weeks) and the indistinguishable *T.b.brucei* (totally harmless to man) had, for many years, been a serious obstacle to progress in defining the nature and extent of the non-human reservoir of this disease, i.e. which of the wild and domestic animals carry the infection, and for how long and which of the tsetse flies transmit it to man.

Earlier last century medical workers in what was then Tanganyika had bravely injected themselves with these T.brucei-group organisms without becoming infected. One classical study was the famous 'Tinde Experiment' carried out at the Sleeping Sickness Research Station at Tinde in western Tanganyika. It examined the continued human infectivity of a *T.b.rhodesiense* strain, taken from man, and cyclically (i.e. by feeding and infecting clean unfed tsetse flies and, when these were positive, feeding them on to other clean animals) through different game and domestic animals for 18 years. At the end it was still infective for man and this quality for 'rhodesiense' was considered immutable. By this time a curative drug (Suramin) had been found which ensured successful treatment thus making human volunteer inoculation acceptable. Local African volunteers were given bicycles or transistor radios and also offered temporary employment at the research centre (e.g. grass cutting and window cleaning) for two years, so that they could be checked to confirm that no recurrence of the infection had occurred. This became very popular and the locals were qeueing up to participate – a week or so in a soft bed, one bout of fever and a few injections seemed a small price to pay for the 'goodies'.

But such were the ethical objections, adding to the difficulties of this laborious research, that only comparatively few human volunteers were ever used. Also, since the scientists could only infect themselves once or twice at most, the true nature and extent of the natural non-human reservoir of this severe ('rhodesiense') form of sleeping sickness in the wild remained unknown. When this new international project started work in the Lambwe Valley, only the one successful isolation and identification of this lethal parasite from a naturally infected wild animal had been that by the Division of Insect-Borne Diseases, Nairobi in 1958 in blood taken from a bushbuck shot in Sakwa, western Kenya) and which quickly put 'Guggi' the recipient into hospital – as mentioned earlier.

Although surveys of the human inhabitants of the valley had been completed, samples of *T.brucei*-type trypanosomes were still being sought and found by Reg (from wild animals), by John the FAO vet., from his 'sentinel cattle' (kept in the fly-infested thicket clearings) and by the entomology team from several of the tsetse flies caught in traps and with a net off bait cattle, and their salivary glands dissected out. Once cattle had been found infected the blood was taken and the sample frozen; the infected animal was then treated and brought up to a holding area in the camp – higher up and away from the valley tsetse hordes.

In an effort to eliminate the tsetse from the Lambwe Valley thickets Dieldrex insecticide was sprayed as an invert emulsion (water droplets surrounded by insecticide solution) firstly by helicopter and later by a low-wing monoplane. Both flew only a few feet above the thicket canopy – working systematically backwards and forwards along pre-marked swathes some 10-12 yards wide. Large square markers mounted on tall poles and held up through the thicket kept the planes on line. As soon as the plane had passed over the indicator the ground team moved quickly to the next pre-marked spot and raised it again quickly while the plane was doing a steep turn, before swooping down and starting the run back with the next swathe in the opposite direction. Refuelling with petrol filtered through chamois leather and with insecticide was carried out by special well-trained teams. The success of this spray activity depended to a large extent upon the droplet size and formulation; their dispersal into and through the canopy was a crucial factor in the success achieved. To avoid the obvious dangers of rising thermal air currents, which began once the land warmed up in the early sunshine and posed a considerable threat to the planes flying only a few feet above the very dense canopy, air-spraying started at first light and continued until late forenoon, when the increasing strength of these rising thermals made such low flying dangerous.

Similar air-spray planes in Botswana flew at night to take advantage of the calm air. These planes were fitted with powerful searchlights pointing both forward and down to light up the canopy. Swathe indicators were illuminated and the pilot and ground staff were in constant radio communication. This seems to have worked well and was popular with the pilots who felt it was even safer than daytime flying (Dr. Giles Leigh-Browne, personal communication). At regular intervals special spraying flights were made over 'jump cards' (Pl.16). These was placed across the swathes, face up and were covered with shiny white paper; and were used to check the number, size and distribution pattern of the droplets, which appeared on the paper as small pink blobs.

Possibly harmful side-effects of the Dieldrex were studied independently and very carefully by Dr. Jan Kuman a Dutch specialist biochemist. He collected samples from wild and domestic animals, from insects and birds, from fish, fish-eating birds and all water sources including the river outlet into the lake. Fortunately no harmful effects were found. Later analysis found that when exposed to sunlight the Dieldrex molecules quickly broke down into more highly toxic and very unstable isomers; fortunately these lasted only an hour or so before disintegrating structurally and becoming harmless. Although the spraying virtually eliminated all tsetse from the thickets on the valley floor, it was unable to reach the steep impenetrable thicket-filled gullies coming down from the Gwembe and Gwassi massifs. Ground spraying and/or fogging were considered but rejected on the grounds of difficulty, expense and with the result being uncertain The inevitable result of this was that a few years later the tsetse population had regenerated from the untouched flies in the gullies and had reoccupied the whole of the valley. This was soon reflected in a growing number of new Sleeping Sickness cases among those visiting and living in the Lambwe Valley.

With the case-finding surveys of the people living in and along the sides of the valley now complete, as mentioned earlier, David Scott asked me to concentrate on characterising the many parasite strains that had been collected from the wild and domestic animals, from wild caught tsetse and from Sleeping Sickness cases. These were all safely stored in the liquid nitrogen cryobank. I started testing them for their behaviour when grown in culture to which different blood and serum samples, different ABO human blood groups and different wild animal serum etc had been added. As normal 'control samples' each strain was grown also in standard cattle or rat serum. We also had in the cryobank some proven *T.b.brucei* strains sent to us by Dr. Raphael Onyango, the Director of the East African Trypanosomiasis Organisation in Tororo, Uganda.

These had been isolated from both wild animals and from domestic livestock. All had failed to infect the human volunteers in whom they had been tested at the EATRO Institute and so were valuable man-tested reference samples. One evening after dinner, when our two children were asleep and Shirley my wife listening to a BBC radio programme, I slipped back to the laboratory to complete the microscopical examination of some blood films from the tests put up earlier that afternoon. In the empty laboratory, and when I had almost completed the wet film examinations, one sample showed only the restless movement of the blood cells and not the vigorously 'kicking' trypanosomes (Pl.15) jostling them, that I expected to see. This was most unusual and when I checked its pedigree I found that it was one of these few man-tested *T.b.brucei* samples that we had borrowed from the EATRO (Uganda) cryobank – as a reference strain. At this stage of the research studies I was, for the first time, incubating known T.b.rhodesiense samples and this control T.b.brucei with my own blood before testing them. This new finding suggested that by exposing these parasites to my own blood in a sterile bottle and incubating them in a 37°C waterbath for one hour, only the human-infective 'rhodesiense' retained their human infectivity. The significance of this, if true, would be like winning the lottery!

Although disturbed in the middle of a Mozart piano concerto and only half-way through his evening whisky, David Scott readily agreed to come with me back to the lab. to check over all my experimental procedures and the results. This we did, very carefully, since he was naturally very sceptical and understandably suspected an error or oversight somewhere. At his suggestion next morning we tested all five man-tested 'brucei' samples together with five 'rhodesiense' samples from recent human sleeping sickness cases. After the vital in-vitro incubation period the mammalian infectivity of these '*rhodesiense*' samples had clearly been retained: by contrast that for the '*brucei*' samples, which had earlier failed to infect volunteers at EATRO, in Tororo, had been lost...

Dr. Ken Willett our former Project Manager, had spent many years on sleeping sickness research working with the famous Tinde and Shinyanga teams in Tanganyika (Drs. Fairbairn and Corson). Now at W.H.O./H.Q.s in Geneva, and on reading the news telexed to him by David Scott, he spent the whole of the Easter holiday in the W.H.O. library – checking all previous records to be sure that this was truly a new and valid finding. Fortunately, it was – and a brief descriptive article was rushed into the W.H.O. Bulletin to claim the priority for this important discovery – which had been sought for nearly

40 years! This was naturally received with much enthusiasm and many Sleeping Sickness researchers immediately set about trying, quite rightly, to find it faulty. Our subsequent applications of this test (which I had named the Blood Incubation Infectivity Test or B.I.I.T.) with *T.brucei* isolates from the wild, gave mostly clear cut negative or positive responses. However, on replicate or triplicate testing, some gave mixed results – some positive- some negative. This was instantly considered by some co-workers as evidence for unreliability of the B.I.I.T.. Conspicuous among these were those who were putting forward other methods of identifying these parasites, i.e. that of displaying and comparing their internal enzyme banding patterns (i.e. isoenzyme characterisation) and looking for successes to secure further research grant funding.

This very elegant technique involves sonicating a homogeneous solution of the trypanosomes in question – to disrupt them and expose their inner components. These include a range of eleven or twelve different enzymes. A well is cut into an agar gel plate and filled with the trypanosome 'soup' and a continuous electric current is passed through it. Rather like the stones on a river-bed the enzymes vary in their specific gravity; the smaller, lighter ones being carried further in the current than those which are heavier.

After a standard time the current is switched off and the agar gel plate is immersed in a blue staining solution. Each of the eleven enzymes then shows up as a distinct band which can be measured and the whole typed. Unfortunately no enzyme banding pattern differences could be found between the '*rhodesiense*' and the more common, non-human-infective '*brucei*'. Although these enzyme patterns were of epidemiological interest they were unable to resolve this problem of identifying the human infective trypanosomes when found in non-human hosts. Only the B.I.I.T. could (and still can) do this.

CHAPTER 17

Exploitation of the B.I.I.T.

Use of the B.I.I.T. to improve understanding – epidemiology and epizootiology – project closes.

The epidemiological value of iso-enzyme characterisation, as it is called, was clearly demonstrated when we investigated a rather severe local outbreak of sleeping sickness later in northern Zambia. Here we were able to trace the origin of the outbreak to an itinerant trader who had recently returned to his home in a small bush village (Kasyasya) in the Luangwa Valley after travelling in other parts of Zambia. We were currently studying sleeping sickness in this village, especially identifying the local wild animals by night drives at the time and since it was some 15 miles through thickish bush and woodland, to save journey time the Kasyasya villagers built us a new hut so that we could sleep over there when late in completing the day's work or doing night drives.

Isoenzyme characterisation of the parasite samples from several different sleeping sickness cases, living in villages within a radius of some 10 miles of Kasyasya were found to have the same rather complicated and unique banding pattern. This was very convincing evidence that this trader, whose infection was of the same pattern, was the source of the generalised outbreak – infecting the tsetse flies in each of the villages that he visited.

We discovered another interesting and possible value for isoenzyme characterisation when we took both blood and cerebral-spinal fluid samples from Sleeping Sickness cases. In some these two samples, isolated separately from the positive case, on the same occasion, were clearly different types – showing marked differences in one, two or sometimes three enzymes, posing the question whether tsetse flies can carry more than one type of trypanosome strain, perhaps one more virulent than the other, or were these two different infections from two different flies. Another interesting question would be – if this case were left untreated and examined again later would we have found both enzyme types in the brain (i.e. cerebro-spinal fluid). As with most investigations – the more one learns the more questions are raised – science is a never-ending study!

In order the better to understand the make-up of these organisms we began studying the long-term behaviour of trypanosome populations, each one grown from a single organism (clone). To make a clone trypanosomes in liquid culture media were serially diluted until only a single one actively moving could be seen in a minute drop of warm saline on a glass slide. This was quickly checked under the microscope by two independent observers, taken up into a small syringe and kept for subsequent long-term study. Further samples were taken at regular weekly intervals – each one being BII tested. This gave valuable, new behavioural information; in essence it showed that both types of the *T.brucei* complex (i.e. '*rhodesiense*' and '*brucei*') were capable of changing into the other and that they were in fact one and the same organism, with a human infectivity potential that was linked with the nature of each of the thousand or more surface coat antigens which the trypanosome changed approximately every 7-10 days.

This is known as antigenic variation, each organism withdrawing the antigenic glyco-protein sheath surrounding it and replacing it immediately with another having a different antigenic identity. .It is this variability that frustrated the efforts to produce a vaccine against this important and deadly disease. Earlier it had been thought that, when first taken up by the carrier tsetse-fly the antigenic repertoire automatically reverted to type 1. If this were so a vaccine produced against, say the first three or four antigenic types, would suffice for the human (or domestic animal) immune response to kill them all off. Unfortunately, this ultimately turned out not to be the case and the first surface antigen types of trypanosomes taken from tsetse flies experimentally infected in the laboratory, were found to vary widely.

At about this time Professor Rudolph Geigy, then Head of the Swiss Tropical Institute in Basel, had been working with his team in and near the famous Serengeti National Reserve in Tanzania. He obtained several *T.brucei* type trypanosome samples from various wild animals and then proceeded to analyse them in detail. Using the cloning technique and our new BII Test, he found clear evidence that when 40% or more of the parasites in an infection were *T.b.rhodesiense* the B.I.I.T. gave a clear-cut positive result: when less it gave an equivocal or clear negative result. With wild animals receiving sometimes hundreds of infective bites a day, the chances of any one animal having a solitary pure infection were extremely remote. Most would be expected to have mixed infections – as

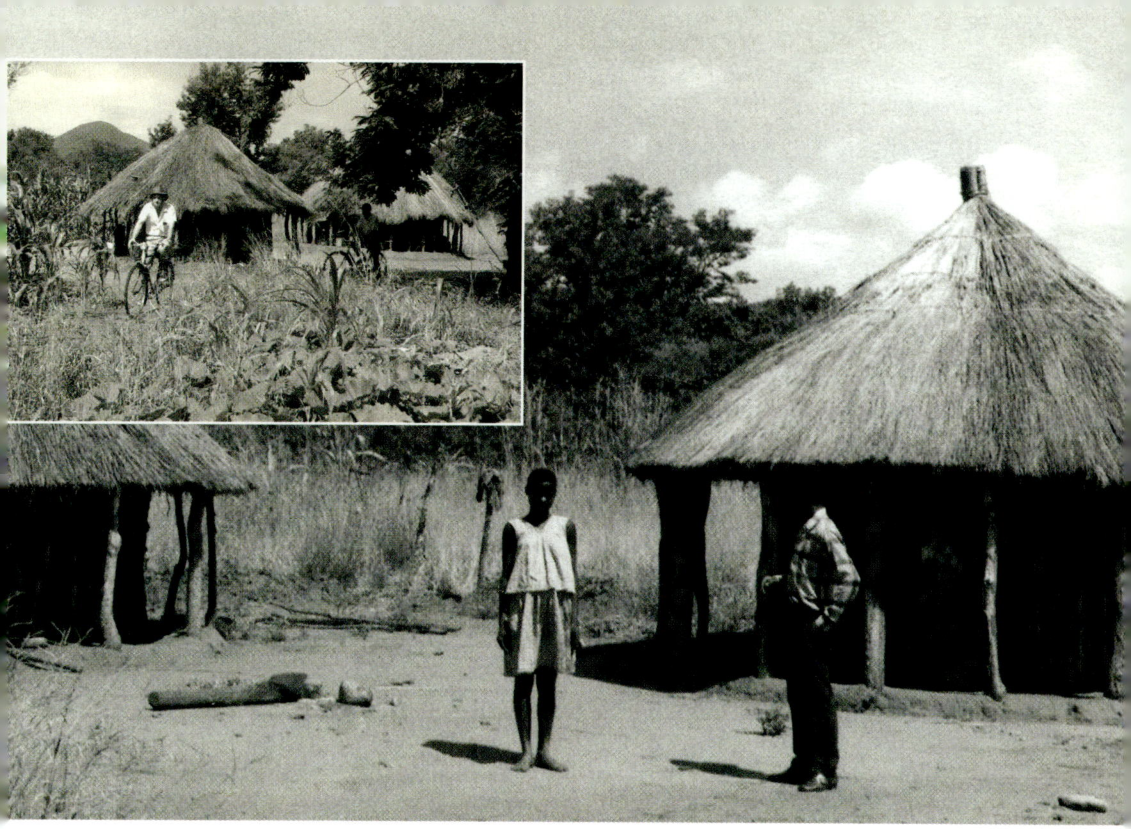

Above: *Plate 22.* Yemi Daka with Salvano in front of her new home
Inset: *Plate 23.* The author and Salvano leaving a deserted bush village, Zambia
Below: *Plate 24.* Collecting capillary blood sample from a trusting donor – Rural Health

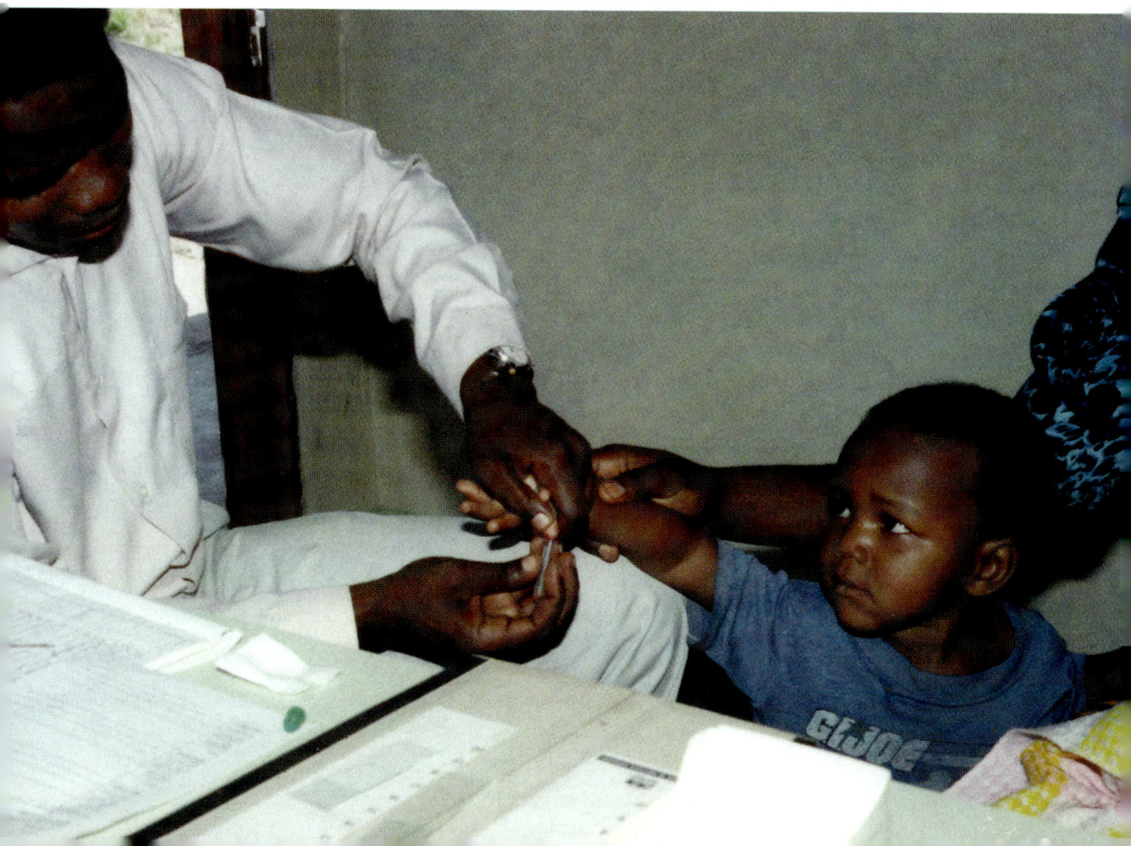

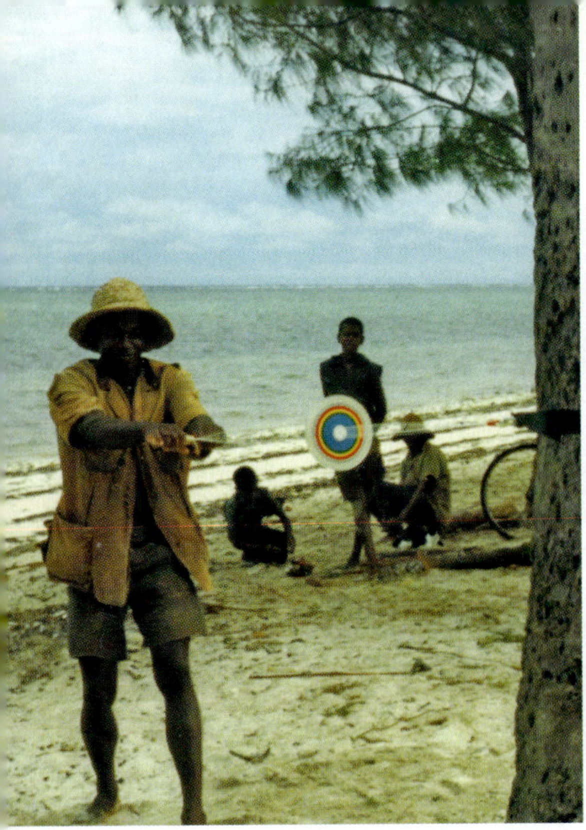

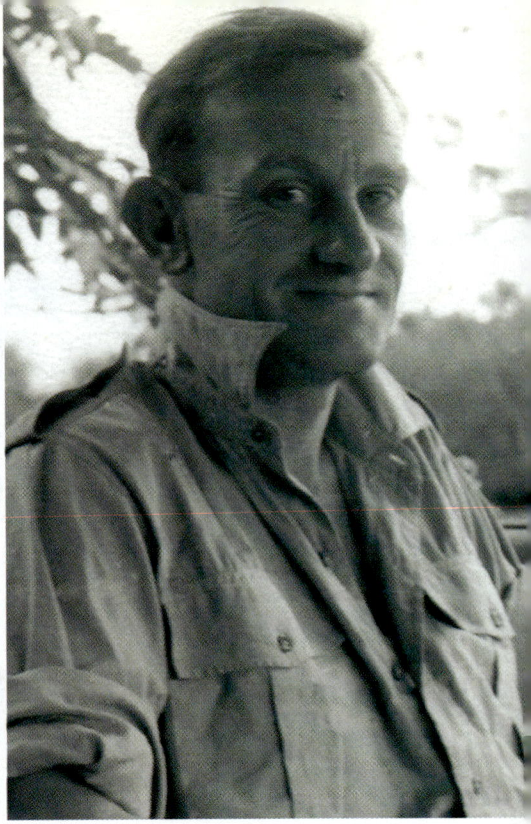

Above left: *Plate 25.* Shark fisherman Simai trying out the Spindoctor string-powered centrifuge to measure anaemia, Makunduchi, S.E. Zanzibar

Above right: *Plate 26.* The Author

Below: *Plate 27.* 'Pablo' with young son Alistair, Dar es Salaam, Tanzania

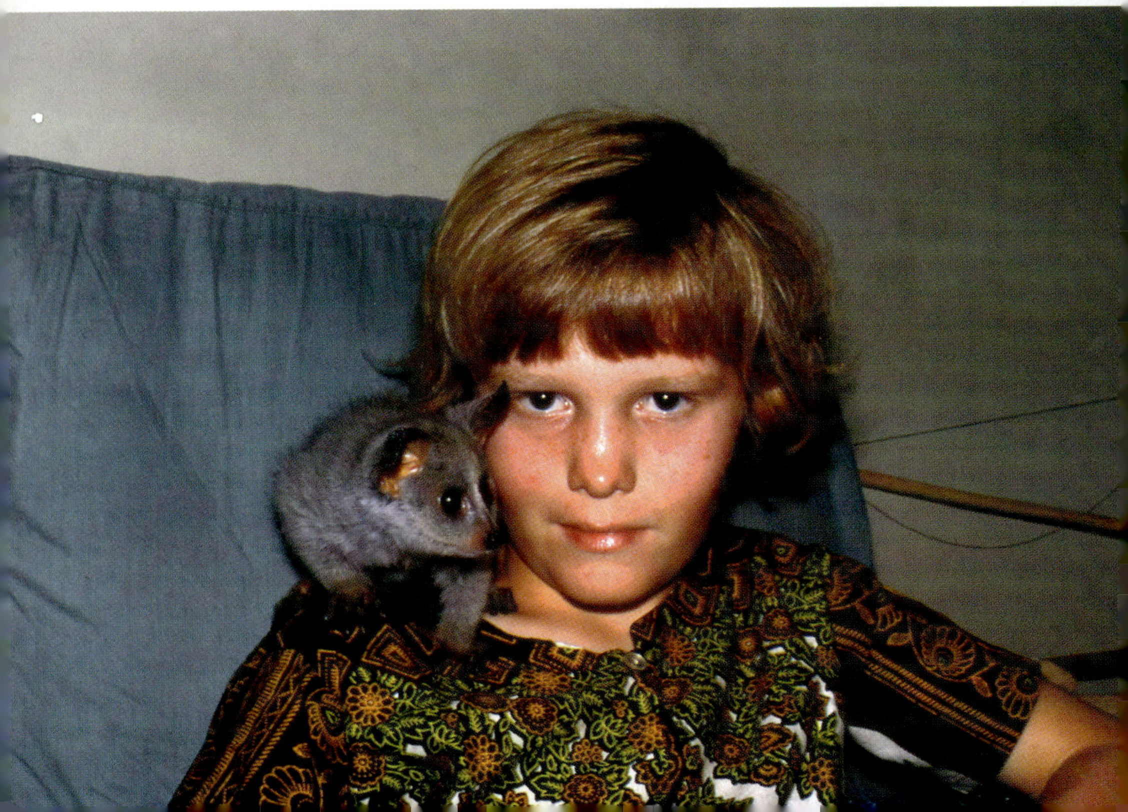

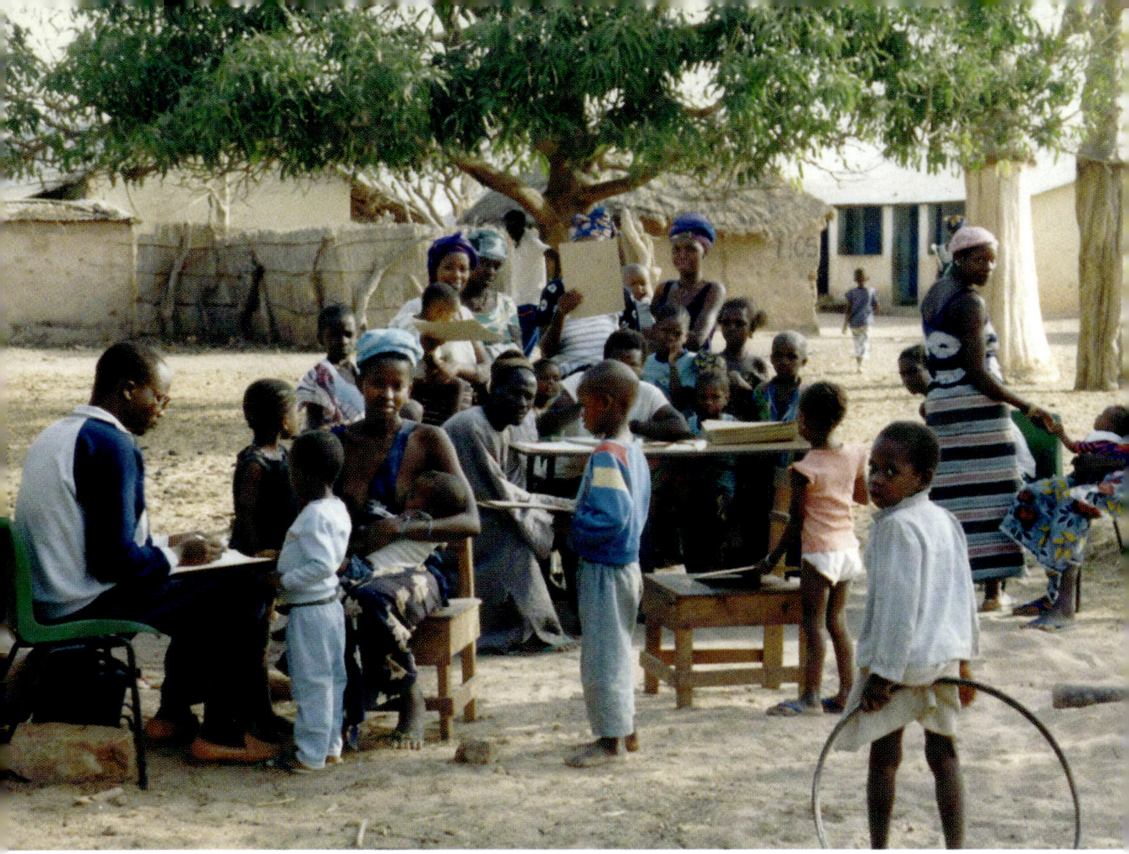

Above: *Plate 28.* Busy field clinic (screening for anaemia and malaria), N. Nigeria
Below: *Plate 29.* Medical assistant taking swab for leprosy diagnosis, Kampumbu, Zambia

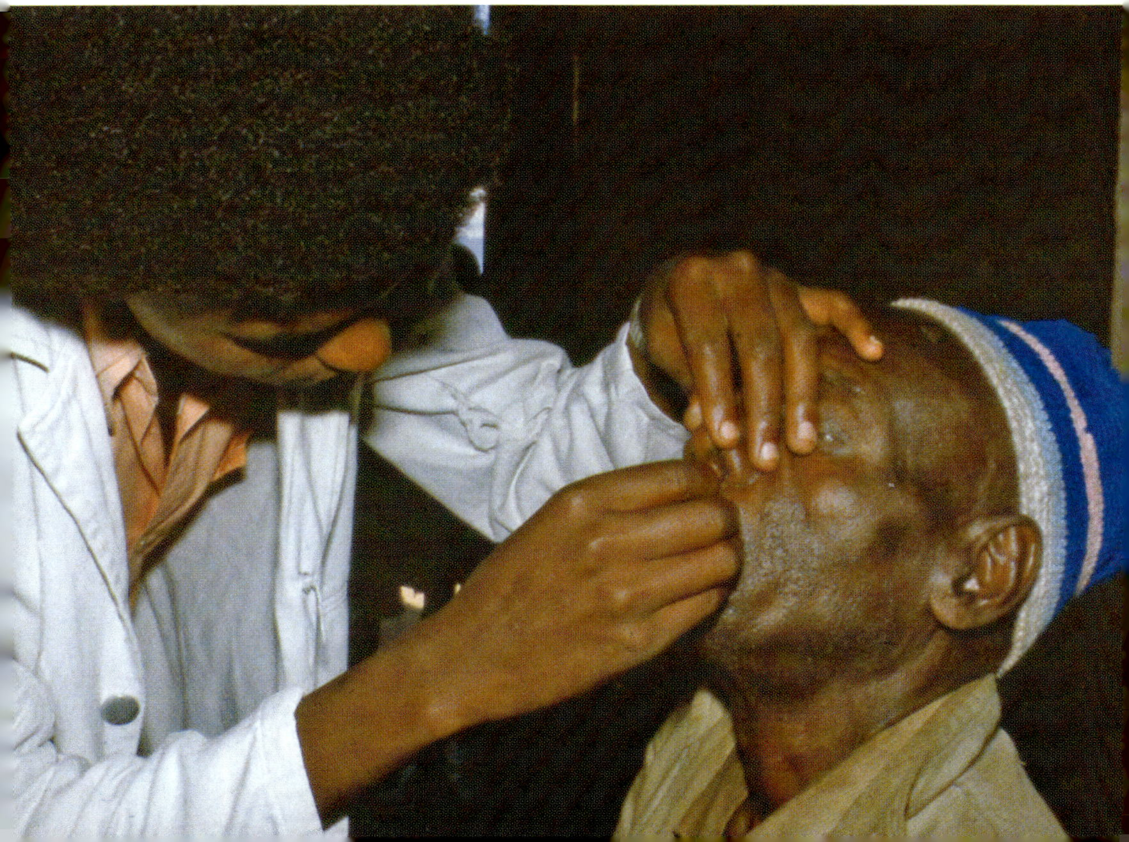

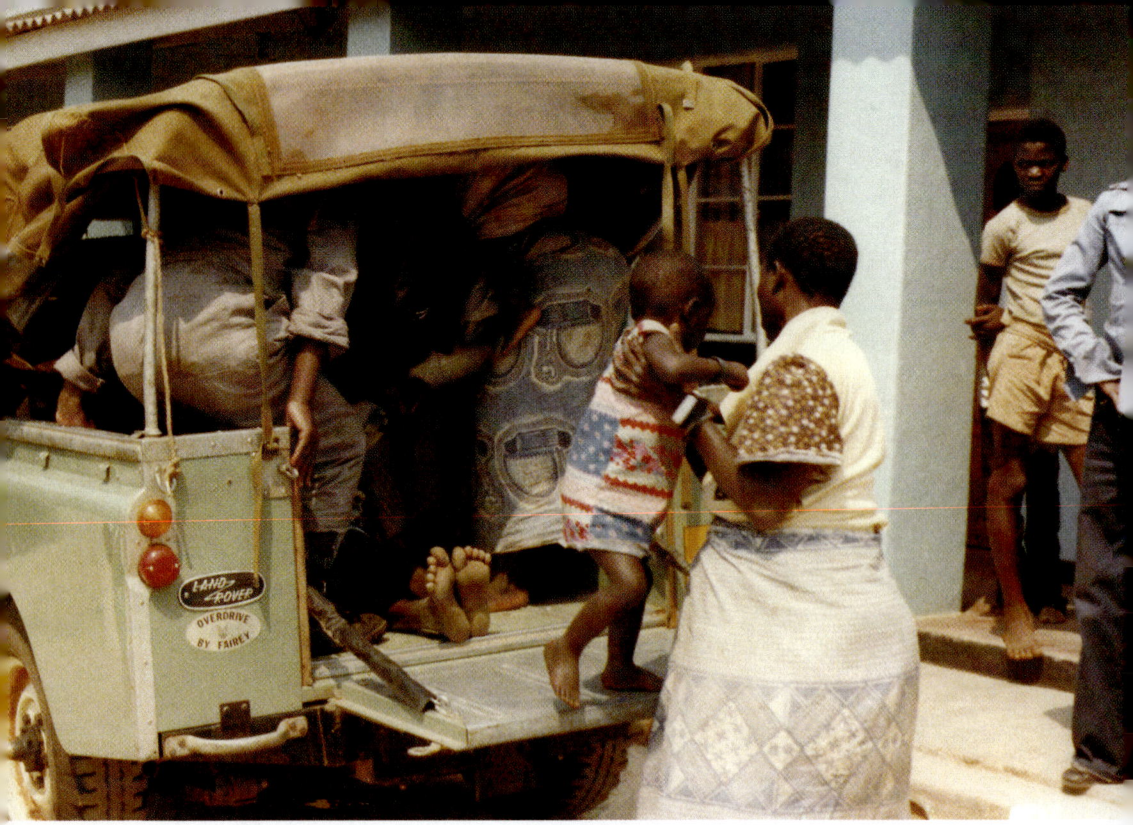

Above: *Plate 30.* Taking sick patients to Chilonga Mission Hospital, Zambia
Below left: *Plate 31.* Technician measures height and weight of cheerful young Zambian
Below right: *Plate 32.* Musician, Kasyasya village, Luangwa Valley, Zambia

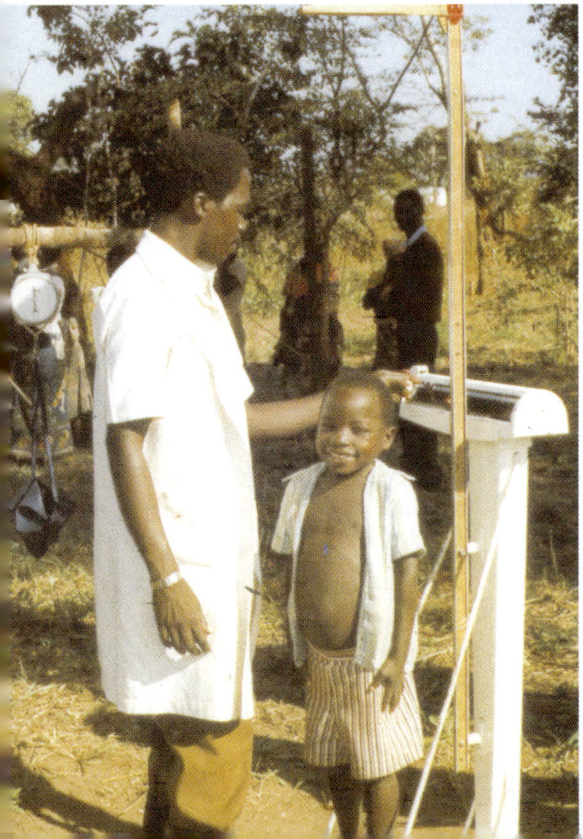

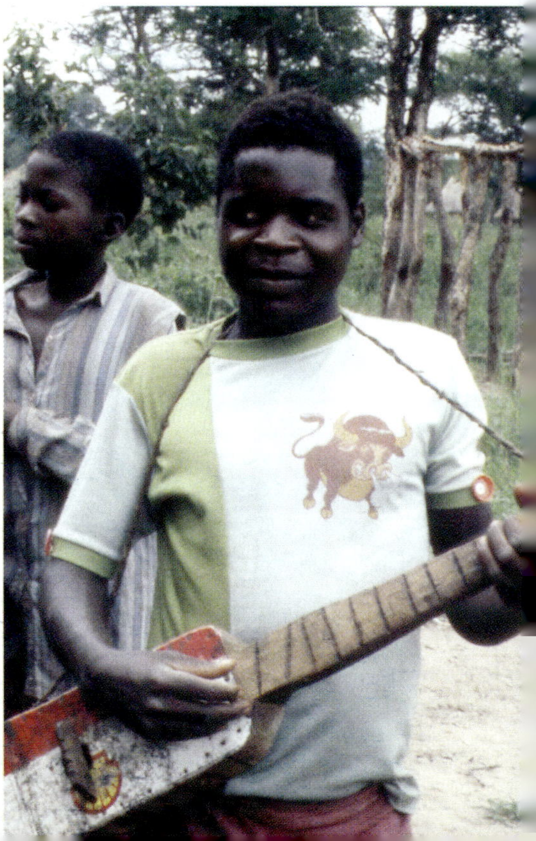

Professor Geigy's Serengeti wild animal surveys and our own clone experiments clearly showed.

To follow up this original finding I was joined by John Robson, our FAO veterinarian and together we began characterising all the *T.brucei* samples that we had acquired. This work was subsequently published and both John & I were officially congratulated on this project success. It was followed by the very successful airspray programme which resulted in (sadly, only temporarily) eliminating the tsetse flies from the main Lambwe Valley thickets.

Most recently, when I had long believed the B.I.I.T. to be dead and buried and to have been merely a 'five-minute wonder' I was delighted to receive an Email from the U.S.A. Dr. Jayne Raper of the Dept. of Medical & Molecular Parasitology, New York University School of Medicine, wrote to say that, more than 30 years later, many scientists were still actively analysing the differentiating factors of the B.I.I.T. – which was still working well.

As the project was coming to its close David Scott suggested that John and I should move to a research institute where we could continue our B.I.I.T. work, since this new test, now proven accurate, could be applied more widely in the many tsetse-infested areas of sub-Saharan Africa. This would at long last identify the wild animal reservoir hosts of this disease and so definitively define its geographical distribution in sub-Saharan Africa. A large number of frozen samples held in cryobanks all over the world, could also be accurately identified and provide a considerable amount of valuable new data to help throw more light on the epidemiology and epizootiology of this hitherto incompletely understood disease.

Unfortunately, at this time, the W.H.O. Regional Director for Africa, had different plans and John and I were split up; John being moved up to Uganda to resume his earlier studies on the tick-borne diseases of cattle (and also suffer severe fear, danger and work restrictions under the infamous Idi Amin regime): I was reassigned to revive what had become a defunct and largely ineffectual malaria research unit in Lusaka, Zambia.

CHAPTER 18

Malaria Research Unit

Resuscitating malaria research in Zambia – asked to survey a malaria-stricken village near Victoria Falls – rewarded with rain and hippo meat.

Athough my reassignment away from Kenya and back to Zambia was initially disappointing, because of my previous training and experience, i.e. with W.H.O. malaria research teams in northern Nigeria and Ghana, this did make some sense. The new buildings for this new unit were presently incomplete and unoccupied, and situated in the grounds of the small psychiatric hospital complex at Chainama Hills. The Chief Health Inspector John Henderson at medical H.Qs immediately saw to the completion of the buildings (which leaked) and of all essential power, lighting and water facilities. There were also three small bungalows in the grounds for senior staff occupation.

The senior staff consisted of 4 Malaria Supervisors, who had been seconded earlier from the almost totally successful Indian malaria eradication programme. Pending their occupation of the new buildings they were temporarily housed in the old hospital morgue – and were happy indeed to see my arrival and their releases from such a macabre working environment! With no proper equipment this at first presented a pretty dismal picture; but, thanks to the dynamic drive of John Henderson, repairs and completion were both soon under way and within a few days the new equipment ordered from W.H.O. began to arrive. This provided the opportunity to start recruiting new staff for the two sections – Parasitology and Entomology – each of which had a separate building with a large laboratory, a small office, wash-room, toilets and a small store. Part of the laboratory was later sectioned off as an insectary. The main building had an office, with store room and toilets and a sizeable lecture room. Transport consisted of three long-wheel-base Landrovers and two caravans. The four Indian staff members were well trained and experienced and were able initially to assist with teaching the new recruits. A general refresher course was started which included, malaria life cycle, survey techniques, patient examination, safe sample collection and processing, accurate record keeping and data consolidation; these were all carefully covered and much time was spent on the all-important aspects of microscopical diagnosis.

The help of the four Indian staff members both in training and in leading the various new research activities undertaken by the unit was invaluable and their help in training certainly accelerated the progress of the new recruits. Soon we were able to start field investigations. The new W.H.O. Landrovers had arrived together with the new microscopes and other key equipment and the staff were keen to make a start – after their long and probably boring period of inactivity.

Two areas were chosen which were considered to be of value, both in terms of basic epidemiological research and collection of accurate base-line data. It was equally important, to identify specific areas in which visitors to Zambia, coming to enjoy the many attractions of this beautiful country, might be unduly exposed to risk of malaria infection. The first unit was established close to the Mpongwe Mission near to Ndola in the Copperbelt. Here the particular scientific attraction was the presence of a special type of malaria vector mosquito – *Anopheles funestus* – which breeds all the year round in the sluggish streams that occurred there and continues transmitting malaria infections endlessly. By contrast the major vector in other parts of sub-Saharan Africa – *Anopheles gambiae* (sensu stricto) – likes only clean water and becomes a very prolific vector of malaria indeed when breeding in the multiplicity of ponds, puddles and gutters and 'borrow pits' that form during the rainy season. This enables it to produce prodigious numbers in a short time and, if able to take blood feeds from people carrying the malaria parasites in the peripheral blood stream, this can rapidly increase the numbers of cases, i.e. within the two weeks or so needed for the parasites to complete their complicated development cycle inside the female mosquito. Once the many thousands of infective forms (sporozoites), have invaded the tubular salivary glands, they are injected into another human when it bites again to take more blood. Blood is needed by the female mosquito for egg production while the male feeds unobtrusively on plant juices.

Most recently geneticists have succeeded in unravelling the genetic code of both the mosquito vector and the most malignant form of malaria (*Plasmodium falciparum*) often called cerebral malaria because of its severe pathology. This unravelling of the genomes has enabled the scientist to make modifications that prevent the development of the parasite inside the mosquito. If this modification can be disseminated and taken up by the Anopheline malaria mosquitoes in the wild, this will constitute the 'magic bullet' sorely needed for the world-wide control of this major killer tropical disease – virtually the 'Holy Grail' of tropical parasitological research!

The second area chosen for research was that of Livingstone in the southern province, because of its continual stream of visitors to see the famous Victoria Falls (Pl.18) or, more properly Mosi-oa-Tunya ('The Smoke that Thunders') its proper and infinitely more attractive local name. At that time the New Intercontinental Hotel directly facing the Falls was understandably very well patronised; it was new, beautifully appointed with excellent cuisine and a fine swimming pool. In the rainy season the mighty Zambezi river is almost a mile wide at the brink and 60 million gallons of water pour over the rock face every minute plunging down 355 ft into the gorge below and continually sending up a dense cloud of spray. Along the shoulders of the rocks facing the falls are footpaths in which the fall-out from the spray trickling down continually has hollowed out shallow steps, the fall-out forming pools which could, at first glance, support mosquito breeding. However, further consideration revealed that the run-off was such that no larvae or pupae could survive in these steps; they would be washed away. Another, even more compelling factor for ruling out malaria risk was the total lack of a malaria reservoir from which any mosquitoes could pick up the infection. Government rules forbade any living accommodation anywhere near the Falls and malaria-carrying mosquitoes feed only at night, when all those working in the area would have gone home.

It was sufficient to ensure that the Intercontinental Hotel (with fully screened and air-conditioned bedrooms) informed all visitors of the very slight risk and make anti-malaria tablets available in the dining room. But this was not to be the end of the affair for, soon after, the unit was joined by another freshly appointed W.H.O. staff member who, immediately on seeing the Falls area, decided unilaterally to undertake special anti-malaria measures. These included cementing all the footpaths opposite the main falls and instituted special vector surveys in the closed areas around them. When the order for many bags of cement and proposals to hire contractors to undertake the work, reached the Ministry of Health in Lusaka I was called there to explain why this was necessary. I pointed out that mosquito breeding on the paths was impossible, because of the high run-off even in the dry season and. more important, there was a total absence of any human nocturnal reservoir. The damage that cementing would cause to the location would constitute a deterrent to visitors, ruining, as it would, the aesthetic appeal of the immediate surrounds of these world-famous Falls... This was accepted and although the proposal was quietly dropped, the MOH requested that a small unit should be left in the area to be on the safe side. This was reasonable and the hospital made a small room available for one of the malaria scouts to use for microscopy to check any suspect malaria cases.

Livingstone itself – some few miles back from the Falls – was a dry and dusty town with one or two touristy hotels and an excellent museum. This had some of Dr. Livingstone's original letters and some of his cothing – incuding the soft cap with its cloth flap at the back to protect the neck... They also had lots of flora and fauna displayed with a beautiful model of the whole of the Falls area and the series of immence gorges with their precipitous sides and most recently the scene of some magnificent white-water rafting. Since my time there the rail-road bridge joining Zambia with Zimbabwe has been the favoured spot for bungee-jumpers – plunging down some 200 ft head-first above the seething white water churning out from the bottom of the Falls.

In the rainy season the Falls are a truly magnificent sight with the mile wide Zambezi river plunging into the deep rocky trough and throwing up a cloud of spray that can be seen for miles. In the early morning this spray throws up millions of multi-coloured diamonds and a rainbow that beggars description! As mentioned earlier from May to October 60 million gallons of water pour over the rock face every minute; but by November, this amount has fallen to 4 million gallons per minute. At this time in the dry season this flow is so much reduced that, with care, one can walk almost right across the top of the Falls – hopping from rock to rock. On the Zambia side, in front of the big hotel, is a fine statue of Dr. Livingstone; it shows him in full stride with his cap on and a shoulder-length sun-flap. Behind this statue (and probably missed by many visitors) is the entrance to a rocky and steep path running down to the 'Boiling Pot' – some 100 yards or so downstream from the Falls. Here the white water rushes past at your feet after surging out through a narrow cleft into the first of three magnificent gorges and, as mentioned earlier these are now much used for white-water rafting. The climb back up from the Boiling Pot is laborious. More worrying in recent years have been reports that this beauty spot has become the focus for muggings and visits there are, or were, discouraged.

The Chief of Mukuni village, some two-three miles from the Falls, sent us word that he would like all his villagers to be examined for malaria. It was then late in the dry season and when we arrived there in the Landrover the Chief was unavailable – busy, we were told, praying for rain to save the villagers' maize and millet crops. We came back again a couple of days later to find that the villagers had just killed a hippo by the Zambezi river nearby and had carried huge chunks of the crudely dismembered carcase back to the village. As we drove in the Chief was up to his elbows inside the hippo remains, covered in blood, with a huge grin on his face and busy carving off huge sices of meat, for those waiting expectantly around him. On seeing us approach he temporarily abandoned his task of chief carcase carver and came over to greet us – his arms red with blood up to the elbows. He grinned his understanding, when I politely refrained from shaking hands, and waved us into his homestead. There had still been no rain and although clearly disturbed at this blatant lack of response by the Almighty to his earlier supplications for life-giving showers, he gave us carte-blanche to carry on with the survey.

We set up a small work-table in the shade of a huge mango tree and started examining and blood-filming all who came, especially the small children who are particularly susceptible to severe malaria infection because of their low levels of naturally acquired immunity. This would grow with the years if they survived further malaria attacks. Most of the infections we found were in the children and these were each treated with chloroquine tablets followed by a large gob-stopper sweet to take away the bitter taste! By the time we had finished it was late afternoon and the large cumulo-nimbus thunder-heads that had been building steadily all afternoon, finally began to make their presence felt. Before we had finished reloading the Landrover they unleashed the first of many shafts of lightning, which were quickly followed by deafening claps of thunder. Then down came the rain, first as individual tea-cup-sized splashes in the sand then soon as a continuous stream of 'stair-rod' dimensions.

The Chief came running up to us beaming broadly and waving an outsized piece of hippo meat and shouting "You have brought the rain to us – thank you – thank you" and handed this gigantic 'Porterhouse' hippo steak to the lads who accepted it gratefully. With a final wave and a grin we set off back along the track which by now was already becoming submerged with the downpour.

Back at base we decided to open another field research unit at Chirundu, just short of the bridge carrying the road the main road from Zambia into Zimbabwe. Mr. Malhoutra, one of the Indian Malaria Supervisors, volunteered to move down to Chirundu to establish and run the new unit. One of the two caravans was placed at his disposal with a Landrover for local running. He was as keen as mustard to have the chance to build such a unit from scratch. Within a couple of months he had built a sizeable laboratory – staff houses and animal pens (to see if local mosquitoes fed upon hosts other than man). The buildings were of sun-dried mud brick, were lime-washed and had gauzed windows. He soon established very friendly relations with the Vlahakis family who ran a large farm along the banks of the Zambezi river, by the bridge, growing pineapples, bananas and many types of vegetables for the Lusaka market.

With his well-trained staff they soon began collecting and characterising the local mosquitoes, producing much valuable baseline data for the area. He soon showed that some of the local mosquitoes were feeding mainly on the 'sentinel' sheep and goats and rarely came to humans. He also provided a valuable reference centre where local people could come for a malaria check when they had fever. The District Hospital was not far away but welcomed the assistance provided by this new specialist Chirundu unit. – especially in the rains when many new malaria cases appeared. The whole team was happy, worked well and collectively did some fine work.

During one of my regular visits there I arranged for Salvano Kanyangala, a well-trained and highly experienced malaria microscopist, to organise an early morning mosquito catch in a local village. Salvano came from this area and besides speaking the local dialect perfectly knew many of the local village people. He chose the village of Chiawa, some 35 miles downstream from the huge Kariba Dam but only five or six from Chirundu – although it meant having to ferry the Landrover across the Kafue river just before its junction with the Zambezi. Having agreed in advance to vacate the sleeping huts just after dawn and without lighting the customary early morning fire (which would have driven out most of the resting mosquitoes), the people greeted us warmly – despite their temporary discomfort! The white catching sheets were laid out in the sleeping huts, the doors closed and windows spaces covered (very few have glass) and the inside then sprayed with a pyrethrum knock-down insecticide. The carefully folded sheets were spread outside on the ground and all insects collected and placed in small specimen tubes. What was most revealing, even horrifying, was the vast army and rich assortment of other creepy crawlies that staggered out from the huts into the bright sunshine; enough to make one realise just how difficult it is for many of these people to enjoy a peaceful night's sleep!

Whilst we were all enjoying a cold bottled drink and just before we started back to Chirundu, a young woman came up to Salvano and asked him if we would look at her sick child in a hut nearby. Once our eyes had adjusted to the dark interior we could see a very small child huddled in a light blanket on the corn-stalk bed. His temperature was 103 degrees and he was almost comatose. We quickly took a small finger-prick blood sample and made two films – one for staining and later microscopy: the second a wet-film for immediate examination. For this we put the microscope on the Landrover bonnet and immediately saw the many eel-like trypanosomes thrashing about among the blood cells. We took the mother and child up to the District Hospital where the lady doctor put the child to bed and found room for the mother to stay. Fortunately it was an early infection and the Suramin injections quickly cured the child. It was the first such case that the doctor had seen in that area; clearly a problem that would have been a fitting and valuable subject for further investigations.

Soon other senior staff members began to arrive. First was David Baldry the entomologist who had been with us in the Lambwe. He had stayed on to complete the very successful fixed-wing airspray trials against the tsetse flies in the valley thickets. David was soon followed by Dr. Sombat Chayabajera a Thai malariologist with a big smile and engaging personality; he had been reassigned from a W.H.O. malaria project in Thailand. A French sanitarian Serge Roche with his wife Magguy arrived soon after from Reunion island. Lastly Annette Fauquex, a young Swiss laboratory technician, was sent out by W.H.O. from Geneva to help with the rapidly expanding training programme.

CHAPTER 19

Sleeping Sickness Epidemic

Investigations at Luembe – visit local Chief and borrow his bicycles

The research programme was now going ahead nicely; the staff were all well trained and safe in their blood-sample collecting, processing, physical examination of patients (oral temperature, pulse, respiratory rate, measuring spleen enlargement), completing the individual questionnaires and making an accurate microscopical diagnosis of malaria. After a little while I was called to visit Dr. Dibue – the W.H.O. Representative in Zambia, who asked me to investigate a suspected outbreak of sleeping sickess in the lower Luangwa valley. Unbeknown to me at the time, this was to have a major influence on my later life.

He said to me "The medical H.Qs statistics section have informed me that a few cases of sleeping sickness are being reported each month from the hospital at Nyimba in the Eastern Province. There is no mention of the location but the Luangwa Valley would probably be a good place to start. Clearly an investigation is needed and, with your recent experience with this disease in Kenya, I would like you to take a small team up there to investigate and take whatever measures you think necessary to bring it under control. How soon could you be ready to leave?" I opted for a quick and immediate reconnaissance of the situation and took two assistants with me, Salvano Kanyangala and Gervazious Tembo, and enough equipment to make accurate on-the-spot examination and diagnoses of suspect cases. This was agreed and two days later we drove up to Nyimba in the Landrover.

The small District Hospital at Nyimba was run by an Indian doctor – Dr. Vaya; it was he who had wisely sounded the alarm when sleeping sickness cases started attending his clinics. He kindly made room for us in his guest-house and, next morning, accompanied us to the wards where he showed us five new cases. We examined them individualy, completing for each a detailed epidemiological questionnaire, e.g. Which village do you live in? How long have you been sick? Where were you bitten – in the bush or in the village? Are there others in your village or living nearby who are also sick like you? Do you go hunting in the bush? Which types of animals live in the bush near your village?

They had one thing in common – they all lived in or regularly visited relatives and friends living in or near the small village of Luembe, situated on the west bank of the big Luangwa river. The bush around Luembe was home to many types of wild animals, many of which were actively hunted for meat.

Millions of years ago, due to a shift in the underlying continental shelf, an enormous fault occurred which split Africa through the Red Sea down to the southernmost part of the continent. This subsidence created the Great Rift Valley system forming the large African lakes and the spectacular scenery of Kenya, Uganda and Tanzania. At the southern border of Tanzania, with Zambia, this rift valley divided. The eastern branch gave rise to Lake Malawi: the western one became the Luangwa Valley, a typical low-lying African river valley carrying the collective rains falling on the surrounding highlands of southern Tanzania and northern Malawi down to join the great Zambezi river at Feira. The valley itself is several hundred miles long with a precipitous western Muchinga escarpment rising to over 2000 ft. The Luangwa river is large, fast flowing and continually changing its course, creating many meanders which it later cuts through to form ox-bow lakes; these subsequently silt up and become lagoons which are attractive both to wildlife and tourists alike' (information based upon the description by Norman Carr in his wonderfully evocative little book about the Luangwa Valley wildlife – '*Valley of the Elephants*' – Collins. London, 1979).

To get to the Luangwa river we had to drive down a narrow, bumpy track which, in places lower down, was much overgrown. It was 40 miles down to the river but, since we had started early, we had time to stop at small hamlets and schools on the way, to examine and to take blood samples from a few who were complaining of fever and body pains. We found two further Sleeping Sickness cases, both showing the highly motile trypanosomes disturbing the red cells. We arranged for these to be sent, with an explanatory note, up to Dr. Vaya at the hospital. Eventually we reached the river and parked the Landrover in the Veterinary Department's special enclosure there. The driver was left there too and given clear instructions about taking any patients that we sent across, immediately up to the hospital – day or night.

The attention of the ferryman, on the far bank, was caught by a loud two-fingered whistle. He waved back, climbed down into the boat and with a long pole started heading slowly up river. A few minutes later he came sweeping down on our side and with practised skill manoeuvred the boat neatly up to the landing platform. The original dug-out canoe had been replaced by a larger and almost certainly much safer plastic boat supplied by the Government. We placed all the equipment and our bedding etc inside and climbed aboard. Using this long punting pole the boatman pushed us slowly up-stream, hugging the bank to avoid the strong current. After some 100 yards he started edging out across the river and, as we began to be caught by the current, hippos suddenly raised their heads on both sides of the canoe (fortunately not beneath us!) and snorted loudly before plunging down again out of sight. The current picked us up, slewed us round and we were soon speeding down the river. With the adept use of the pole the ferryman turned us à la moment critique and we drifted sideways into the opposite bank, clambered up and started unloading.

Where we arrived the Luembe Rural Health Centre was close by and several of the many children from the nearby school took time off from their studies to come out and inspect these new and unexpected arrivals. They were soon pressed into service – carrying the equipment and our bedding upto the Health Centre. George Banda, the resident Medical Assistant, came out and greeted us warmly. Later, when he heard the purpose of our mission, he was truly overjoyed that someone had, at last, come to do something about the sleeping sickness epidemic in a cluster of small hamlets some 5-6 miles away to the west of his Health Centre. He made space for our luggage in his store-room and we erected our camp beds and rigged mosquito nets on the wide verandah. Welcoming cups of tea were soon produced – which surprised me a little, knowing how difficult it must be to get such items from the nearest shops in Nyimba, more than 40 miles away.

The Luembe outbreak area lies about 30 miles east of the junction between the Lunsemfwa and Lukusashi rivers – just above their junction with the Luangwa river. The climate is hot and humid, the vegetation mainly mixed with mopane and acacia woodland and with isolated ranges of forest-clad hills (covered with Brachystegia-Isoberlinia woodland) rising to heights of 3,250 ft amsl. George told us that almost all cases came from this cluster of small hamlets. He had been seeing them in small numbers for some time but recently the numbers began to increase and he rightly feared that a major outbreak was already under way. One aspect that made matters worse was that some of the cases he cycled out to examine fled into the bush on his arrival so that he was unable to catch up with them. We slept well that night in the cool night air and the soothing sound of the river. Next morning George took us to meet the Senior Chief of Luembe. He was a short stocky man with a huge smile; he greeted us warmly, invited us into his well furnished hut and offered us tea and bananas. There was no evidence to suggest that this particular area had been an active focus of sleeping sickness in recent times and he confirmed that this disease had not been a problem among his people since his arrival there in 1946. However, late in 1970 villagers in Kanukawanga and Chimanganya hamlets began to fall sick and, refusing to heed his advice for them to report to the medical centre for treatment, they finally became drowsy, unable to walk and died. He said that he, too, had been one of the early cases and had been successfully treated at the Nyimba hospital.

With the exception of the thirty-three goats belonging to the Chief (thirteen of which had trypanosome infections – but only one of which was a *T.b.brucei* type), there were no other domestic animals in the area; this was almost certainly due to the very heavy tsetse fly presence. But wild animals abound and are hunted vigorously by most of the men-folk. Some wild animal species are known to carry sleeping sickness parasites in their blood for long periods without showing any evidence of disease. For this reason they are important reservoirs of the infection and are particularly dangerous if they are infected when they come close to human dwellings and the local tsetse flies feed upon them and start transmitting the infection rapidly to the villagers in and around the settlements. The transmission cycle changes immediately from the game-tsetse-man to the far more dangerous man-tsetse-man i.e. epidemic conditions. Agricultural activity outside the immediate confines of the villages is minimal and the surrounding bush thickets are often allowed to grow right up to the huts. That contact between villagers and the tsetse flies had become very high was evidenced later when flies were biting us inside the villages – sometimes even when examining villagers inside their huts.

The Chief offered maximum cooperation which included the use of three (Flying Dragon) Chinese bicycles which had clearly seen better days but which, after some remedial work with pliers, screwdriver and pump, were fine. He acknowledged the fear of this disease among the villagers and the reluctance of some to be examined or go up to the Nyimba Hospital for treatment. Unfortunately George was not able (or allowed by medical law) to provide the front-line treatment for the early stage of this killer disease – when the parasites are still only in the blood and lymph channels and can be easily and completely cured. After about a month with this type of sleeping sickness the parasites finally penetrate the 'blood-brain barrier' and multiply in the cerebro-spinal-fluid, the effect of their waste products on the delicate membranes in the brain producing the later stage symptoms – sudden sleeping (sometimes with unchewed food still in the mouth), tremors, slurred speech and inability to walk without falling and ultimately death.

It was a sad and not fully understandable fact that use of the drug Suramin (Antrypol) which was then, and is still, virtually 100% successful in clearing the blood and lymphatics of trypanosomes and keeping them clear for more than three months, is banned for use in the field, away from the hospital. This is due primarily to the possibility of dangerous side-effects shown by a few patients (the incidence of this adverse reaction has been estimated at between 1 in 2000 to 1 in 4,500). To avoid this it is recommended to give a test dose of 0.2 g first and, if no adverse reaction is seen within a few minutes, this is followed later by the main injections. It seems remarkable that permission for trained Medical Assistants to treat confirmed sleeping sickness cases in the field with Suramin, in this type of epidemic situation, is not forthcoming. Logic suggests that it should be standard practice; it would be particularly effective in eliminating an incipient sleeping sickness epidemic by rapidly reducing the human reservoir of infection since its efficacy in keeping patients free from further early stage blood and lympatic infections can last for up to six months.

Against the possibility of an adverse reaction occurring (however serious) must be balanced the 100% fatalities that must be expected when sleeping sickness epidemics occurs in such remote rural communities where the appropriate curative treatment is not immediate available and where the nearest hospital is nearly 50 miles away – across a major river and difficult terrain. It should be mandatory to ensure that all known sleeping sickness foci, active or quiescent, should have this drug available at the nearest Rural Health Centre and the Medical Assistant given permission to use it as required.

Another very serious problem often preventing early and accurate diagnosis (which greatly facilitates the more efficaceous early accurate treatment) is the lack of more appropriate diagnostic instruments, notably a good quality microscope, that can be used where neither generated electricity nor access to a good vehicle battery are available. Good quality microscope is a *sine qua non* for confirming the diagnosis of most of the major communicable diseases.

CHAPTER 20

Finding Sleeping Sickness Cases

Luembe – the sad story of Yemi Daka – a star performance by Medical Assistant George Banda

The next morning, mounted on our newly acquired bicycles, we set out from the Rural Health Centre (RHC) accompanied by George Banda the medial assistant, to visit the outbreak area villages – cycling easily along the smooth earth footpaths running through the thickly forested woodland and thickets. As all cross-word puzzlers know sleeping sickness (or African trypanosomiasis – which not all can spell and few can pronounce properly!) is carried and transmitted to humans by tsetse flies which are motivated mostly by movement. Cycling along the paths we soon attracted a sizeable following swarm, which stopped and settled in large numbers, mostly on the surrounding vegetation, whenever we stopped; only very few were biting. These were the well-known female-seeking males – fortunately more interested in chatting up the local 'tsetse talent' than wasting time on us. George led us into the nearest hamlet; apart from one elderly woman it was totally deserted and had the air of having been abandoned. The bush thicket had been allowed to encroach up to the edge of this village and it was full of tsetse flies which started attacking us. Tsetse dislike crossing open spaces but when the bush is allowed to grow right up to the village edge they can feed readily on the inhabitants – creating the typically epidemic Sleeping Sickness conditions recognised by the equal numbers of women and children occurring with those of adult males among the cases.

This lone inhabitant, too, was clearly very ill but was still trying to pound some few maize cobs in a mortar for the next meal, but with hardly enough strength left to lift the heavy wooden pestle. She was virtually incoherent, mumbling and crying to herself and strongly resisted any attempt by George to question or examine her, despite his quiet reassurances. While we were trying to question her – she suddenly dropped the wooden pestle and ran away and hid in a nearby hut. We decided that the kindest thing was to leave her in peace and so cycled back to Luembe. The following day we returned to find the hamlet totally deserted with no sign of the woman; the Chief later told us that she had run away into bush and had died.

We went on to visit the next hamlet Vuno which was again almost totally deserted. There was one middle-aged woman (Margret Phiri) (Pl.19) on the verandah grinding millet flour for the evening meal. She complained of feeling unwell and, when we examined her blood, we found the actively motile parasites jostling the red blood cells. We spent a long time trying to persuade her to let us take her to the Nyimba hospital where she could be treated – otherwise she would die. She promised to talk about it with her husband when he returned from harvesting his crops, and would come to Luembe to seek the advice of the Chief. We cycled back to Luembe, washed away the dust and travel fatigue and prepared our beds and mossie-nets on the verandah for the night, before enjoying the evening meal of 'posho' (maize-meal porridge) and some tinned stew, beautifully cooked on the ubiquitous charcoal stove and washed down with a tin or two of cool refreshing lager brought with us for the occasion. The tins of beer were kept cool immersed in a net dipped into the river and well secured to a nearby tree! Later that evening a big storm blew up with vivid shafts of lightning, crashing thunder-claps and wind-driven rain. This effectively drove us to abandon the cool of the verandah and seek less comfortable shelter huddled together inside.

Next morning, though still a little bleary-eyed we started the investigation but while we were getting the equipment packed on to the bicycles the Chief approached leading a young woman who had a small boy, named Cosmas Mtonga, in her arms. She wanted us to examine him since he was clearly comatose and was having convulsions. When quickly examined in the Health Centre his temperature was 104 degrees Fahrenheit and to check whether sleeping sickness or malaria, we took a drop of blood on to a glass slide, added on a thin glass cover-slip and put it under the microscope, Immediately we could see many trypanosomes wriggling vigorously about among the red blood cells – acute sleeping sickness. We whistled to the driver and waved to him to stand by for a new patient. The mother and child were lowered into the ferry-boat, transferred to the Landrover on the other side and immediately rushed off up to the Nyimba Hospital where the driver handed the mother and child to the care of Dr. Vaya, together with my explanatory note. Sadly, the little boy survived the two-hour drive up to the hospital only to die some 10 minutes after admission. Perhaps had we been able (i.e. allowed) to give the first Suramin injections at Luembe he might just have survived – we shall never know.

It was the sudden local increase in the number of Sleeping Sickness cases diagnosed in the Nyimba hospital, most in the late (brain-infected) stage of the disease, that finally rang the alarm bells. With proper monthly surveillance visits to all of these outlying village communities and schools, such outbreaks would be discovered at a much earlier stage and the appropriate action taken to treat and temporarily remove such patients from the vicinity – to reduce the human reservoir of infection. Unfortunately, the lack of suitable transport, to enable the health service staff to reach these distant communities, and the lack of solar-powered diagnostic tools that could be used perfectly well in the absence of electricity, together prevent the early diagnosis and treatment of the major communicable diseases and give early warning of incipient epidemics. Although, according to the Chief, there was no evidence to suggest that the Luembe area had been an active focus for Sleeping Sickness in recent times, Dr. K. Willett, one of the early pioneers researchers into this disease, when reviewing the history of this disease in Zambia, describes how, soon after the first cases were found early last century, several more were reported in the Luangwa Valley – near Nabwalia and Hargreaves. These crossing places of the river were closed in 1910 due to the high risk of infections there; Hargreaves is only 2-3 miles upstream from Luembe..

Because of the reported existence in that area of symptomless sleeping sickness cases, discovered by Drs. Ross & Blair in what is now Zimbabwe, with the need to examine as high a proportion of the local population as possible, our diagnostic surveys were carried out on a village-by-village basis, the few people still living in these affected hamlets being carefully examined and small blood samples taken for immediate on-the-spot microscopical examination. While villagers were being examined Salvano and Gervazious, aided by one of the Chief's messengers, were sampling the local tsetse population – to identify the species responsible for the outbreak. This was done by walking about in the surrounding bush and hamlets carrying a large dark blue blanket draped over a long stick on their shoulders. Salvano walked beside them catching the tsetse as, attracted by the movement and colour, they settled on the blanket and were swept up in a small hand-net. Many were caught in this way – all of them the thicket-loving *Glossina morsitans morsitans*.

Earlier several of the villagers from Kanukawanga and Chimanganya had confirmed what the Chief had told us, how, towards the end of 1970, many people had sickened and died in these hamlets – refusing to attend either the Rural Health Centre or go up to the hospital for treatment. It seems that these were never officially reported or investigated but, since many of them were said to have been sleeping excessively and were totally incapacitated before death, they were all probably terminal Sleeping Sickness cases. Kanukawanga was the next hamlet we visited. We arrived to find the place totally deserted and re-invasion of the bush well advanced – some huts already disappearing from view (Pl.20); only a few old cooking pots, and circles of stones where fires had been bearing silent witness to its having been home to several families; the swarms of tsetse flies being the only remaining inhabitants. We continued on to the next village – Chimanganya (Pl.21). When we entered the Headman came to greet us and after giving us a general overview of the virtual destruction of the village, related a poignant story about one of his villagers – Alani Daka. When first sick he refused to go to the RHC or hospital for treatment. He moved with his parents to the village of Penyesani – only a mile away from the Luembe Health Centre – where he stayed for several weeks, sick and unable to walk, before he was carried in a pitiful condition and too late, to the Nyimba hospital 40 miles away, where he died soon after admission.

Having examined the Headman who was healthy enough, we next looked at an elderly man sitting in the shade of a large tree. Senti Ngandu came from the village of Singwendi and had come to visit his sister Zelina. When questioned he said that he had general body pains and a slight headache but otherwise felt well. Unfortunately on examination trypanosomes were clearly seen disturbing the red cells and when we explained that, although he felt well, he too had the infection, he accepted to be taken up to the hospital for treatment. While we were examining him a muscular young man was harrowing his maize 100 yards or so away. When we hailed him he waved, dropped his hoe and came across to join us in the shade of the tree. This young man, Blackson Njobvu, was powerfully built, looked in very good health and smiled in disbelief when we asked him if he felt at all sick. We took a blood slide as a precaution for examination and saw that he too had the infection. Although he was at first reluctant to go to hospital he accepted to accompany old Senti Ngandu when we explained that, without treatment, he would die.

He waved us farewell and walked away back to his harvesting, leaving old Senti to enjoy the cool shade of the tree. We carried on through the hamlet, noting already that a number of huts were deserted and showing signs of dereliction, but stopped when we saw a young woman walking towards us. She was Yemi Daka aged 22 years and recently married; her husband she said was away working on his 'shamba' (cultivated plot) but would be back the following day. Yemi was the younger sister to poor Alani Daka, who had died so wretchedly earlier.

On our initial examination she was completely symptomless – no pains, no fever, no headache and said she felt well. When I started to examine her blood under the microscope I saw nothing abnormal at first, and my hopes rose; but when I continued the search (just to make sure) once again I found one or two trypanosomes characteristically wriggling among the red cells. We explained the need for her to be treated in hospital as quickly as possible, before the infection became worse and much more difficult to cure. Yemi replied that she wouldn't go up to the hospital but said that we could treat her there in the village. I explained that by law we were not allowed to inject this drug (Suramin) away from the hospital but we would take her up to Nyimba in the Landrover – together with old Senti Ngandu and Blackson both of whom she knew. But she was adamant and still refused. When I told her that without the injection she would die Yemi replied that in that case she would die here in the village among the few remaining members of her family and friends. Seeing the camera slung over my shoulder Yemi asked if I would please take a photo for her and I immediately agreed. She explained that her newly acquired husband had just finished building two new huts for them to live in and she wanted a picture taken of her, with Salvano, standing proudly in front of them. She led us a short way through the bush to a small clearing where there were two beautifully built and newly-thatched huts. She stood in front of them with Salvano whilst I took the picture (Pl.22). Copies were sent later but whether they reached Yemi in time I do not know. However, some little time after we had finished the survey and returned to Lusaka, Yemi died. This was quite unnecessary for, had we been allowed to give her the life-saving Suramin injection and left more supplies with George Banda for follow-up treatment, she would still be alive today to bring up the family which she was looking forward to raising. Not being medically trained I must confess that I cannot understand why a drug that will cure virtually 100% of early sleeping sickness infections and immediately and drastically reduce the infection reservoir, cannot be given in the field situation by suitably trained rural health workers. It is still the first drug of choice today for the early haemo-lymphatic Sleeping Sickness infection. That a very few patients so treated may have an adverse reaction to its use is surely outweighed by the fact that virtually 100% of those not treated or cannot get to hospital to receive the injections, will die a degrading and unpleasant death. Fit as young Blackson

Njobvu certainly seemed to be, knowing him to have the infection we requested George Banda to make sure that both he and Senti Ngandu went up to the Nyimba hospital. They eventually did so but, sadly, left it too late and both died soon after admission.

The collective failure of the villagers to cut back the bush, to keep the tsetse flies away from the village, their persisting fear of this disease and of hospitalisation for treatment and the almost totally inadequate Primary Healthcare delivery, allow this situation to persist. Several of the trypanosome samples were carefully harvested, frozen in liquid nitrogen (-196°C.) and transferred to the cryobank at the London School of Hygiene & Tropical Medicine. It is hoped that further studies on these parasite samples may finally reveal why they remain asymptomatic for so long in their human hosts, before finally causing their deaths. When we last met the Senior Chief of Luembe he was in the process of moving what was left of his community up-river where they would establish a new settlement called New Ambo.

Towards the end of this particular field study we had an excellent and unexpected opportunity to witness, at close hand, the expertise of George Banda, the Medical Assistant at the Luembe Rural Health Centre. With no electricity, no serviceable microscope, very few chemotherapeutic drugs and little clinical equipment it would be easy to underestimate the competence of such rural health workers to deal with some of the day-to-day problems. On our last visit to Chimanganya (Pl.23) we arrived back at the Luembe RHC to find George in the middle of holding an 'Under-5s' clinic. The entrance to the Centre was blocked by some 30 or 40 mothers – each with a child slung high up on the back with a shawl knotted at the front.

As he heard the sound of our approach George started to come out to greet us – the gathering of mothers moving back en masse to allow him to do so. A mother at the back, too slow to give way and pushed backwards by the moving crowd, lost her balance and fell back. By cruel chance the baby's head struck a sharp edged rock protruding from the ground which split the skin and made a nasty looking wound. Clearing the crowd with a sweep of his arm George disappeared inside and quickly came out again armed with what he needed to deal with the problem. Taking a new safety razor blade from its envelope and with a small antiseptic swab he cleansed the wound and, holding the razor blade between finger and thumb, with a few deft strokes shaved both sides of the wound, leaving it open and ready for stitching. This, too, was quickly accomplished, the wound area swabbed again and a plaster added. Not once did the baby cry while this was being done. Masterly!

It was a sad fact that we had been able to save the lives of only a few of the villagers. Clearly the lack of regular and effective medical surveillance, the very poor (virtually non-existent) diagnostic facilities at the Luembe Rural Health Centre (with no reliable microscope, no front-line curative drugs for sleeping sickness or permission to use them) exacerbated by the villagers' fear of this disease and their resultant reluctance to go up to hospital for treatment, prevented a satisfactory resolution of this problem and will probably continue to do so while those unhappy circumstances remain.

CHAPTER 21

Anti-malaria Drug Trial

Farewell Luembe – a school fire-dance – see myself in school text-book – demonstration of elephantiasis to villagers – an anti-malaria drug trial in school-children – visit the Kariba Dam.

Since it was nearly dark when we crossed back over the river from Luembe and drove up to the main road, we decided to stop overnight at a local school. This we did regularly when surveying rural communities – especially when carrying out regular medical checks on the school-children for malaria. This made things easier and, once we had the headmaster's O.K., with the classroom now empty we had plenty of space for our beds and for cooking – without disturbing anyone. As we first approached the school we saw that the staff and children were having what turned out to be a practice for the forthcoming Independence celebrations. There was a huge bonfire with sparks sailing high up into the darkening evening sky. Children were practising their dancing to the music supplied by the impromptu band – one very small boy with a home-made one string-guitar: the other beating out an irresistible rhythm with two sticks on an empty oil drum. All children were clearly thoroughly enjoying themselves – as were we. Using my small portable radio-cassette recorder I taped some 30 minutes of this 'concert'.

At the end I played it back to them – to their great delight and many started dancing again! As I write this, many years later, I still have that cassette and still find that simple music extremely evocative – with eyes closed I can still see the sparks rushing up into the night sky and the frenzied dancing of the children. But there was one special surprise waiting for me as I accepted the headmaster's offer to use his office as a bedroom for the night. I went along to his office to find my camp-bed already set up and the pressure lamp hissing merrily on the side table. To one side of the room were kept the racks of school text-books and, responding instinctively to the urge to look at some of them, I noted one on geography of England written by a Mary Temple (a distant relative I believe of the former Archbishop of Canterbury). It had numerous black and white pictures, of different scenes and buildings in the U.K. As I started to riffle through the pages I suddenly got the shock of my life – I was looking at a picture of myself! I was with four other young men all with rucksacks, nailed boots and hill walking gear, standing together having just emerged from a local shop. The caption read... "English hill walkers at Ambleside, Lake District, setting out for the mountains". I remembered the occasion clearly since, some 20 years earlier, when finally released from the wartime forces, my friends and I were setting out for our first experience of hill walking – and we had just been stocking up with food before setting out. A strange coincidence!

On the way back next day we turned off the main road just before Rufunsa and drove some 25 miles of very challenging, sometimes frightening, road which would have done justice as a river bed. It led to a village called Shikabeta – on the bank of the Lunsemfwa river some 20 miles or so above its junction with the Lukusashi – both rivers then flowing south to join the Zambezi at Feira. The reason for the visit was to ascertain a report that this was a focus of the parasitic worm *Wuchereria bancrofti* – the lymphatic filarial worms which, when transmitted by nocturnally biting mosquitoes, become mature, coil up and come to lie in and eventually block the lymph drainage channels – usually those in the legs, scrotum and breasts. This leads to local tissue proliferation which, with repeated infections over time, can become massive and causing gross swellings – known commonly as 'elephantiasis' or 'big leg disease'. This form of the disease is of particular interest since it exhibits 'nocturnal periodicity'. The infective larval worms coming into the blood only at night when the mosquito vectors are biting. Having organised our overnight sleeping arrangements, just before midnight we drove the Landrover into the middle of the 'village green' and set out the microscope, lancets (for blood taking), glass slides and the pressure lamp under the stars. To attract the villagers to come for examination I also put the radio-recorder on the bonnet, put in the recorded cassette of the children singing and dancing and turned up the volume to maximum. The recorded 'concert' was well received since most of the villagers knew the songs and were singing the words as they approached; the light, the music and the children singing well-known local songs attracting them in to the Landrover.

From each a little finger-prick drop of blood was taken on to a glass slide, a thin glass cover-slip added to spread the blood and the sample then examined at 200 magnifications. Whenever one sample showed the microfilarial worms twisting about among the red cells the recipient was invited to see his or her parasite, although not all were keen to do so!

The drug diethylcarbamazine ('DEC') is used to kill these immature blood forms that are picked up by the biting mosquitoes, while Suramin is effective in killing most if not all of the residual adult worms in the deeper tissues. This brief stop-over visit was valuable, both for confirming the presence of Bancroftian filariasis in this small focus but also in making the villagers aware of the problem and also stimulating their acceptance of subsequent treatment. This would be available during the regular monthly outreach clinics carried out by the doctors and staff of the local Mission Hospital near Rufunsa – on the main Lusaka-Chipata road close by.

Soon after our return to Lusaka I had a surprise phone call one Saturday morning from the Ridgeway Hotel where Professor George Nelson was staying there together with Dr. Hugh Jolly, a well-known paediatrician at the Charing Cross hospital in London and radio broadcaster. Apart from a courtesy call at the Ministry of Health and University on business they had a couple of spare days and wondered if it would be possible to see something of Zambia during this brief stopover. The Sunday was spent sailing at the Kafue dam; Hugh Jolly was a keen sailor and his solid build made him an excellent crew to sit out with the jib sheet in the strong afternoon winds. During dinner that evening, at the hotel, George Nelson asked if it would be possible to visit the new Kariba Dam, now very near completion. I thought that, because of the tension then obtaining between Zambia and Zimbabwe, the dam would be very heavily guarded and we could be stopped at any of the many armed road-blocks en route; however, we decided to try.

The first obstacle came when we arrived at the Bailey bridge over the Kafue river. Two soldiers armed with automatic assault rifles approached the car and, as they did so, Hugh Jolly began to open the car door to get out. He quickly decided that discretion was the better part of valour when the muzzle of an AK47 was thrust almost into his face. "We will tell you if and when we want you to get out" said one of the armed heroes. I quietly explained that these were two high-ranking British medical officials who would be visiting President Kaunda in Lusaka before flying back to Europe.

This immediately elicited a far more friendly reaction and we were then given explicit instructions as to how to get to the Kariba dam and they said that they would phone ahead to let other road blocks know that we were coming. They both then saluted smartly and wished us a happy journey We passed three or four other roadblocks en route without any fuss and at the approach to the dam, parked the car and walked halfway across the top of the dam to the barrier with Zimbabwe. There was no other soul in sight – we had the place to ourselves. The Kariba dam was certainly very impressive and was already spilling water in a huge jet from the almost full Lake Kariba behind. In the dry season of course the various pools downstream along the river bank would breed many millions of mosquitoes mostly *Anopheles gambiae* which prefer the cleaner still water. During the rains however the frequent releases of spill-water flowing rapidly down river would flush all of these away. Villages to the east, on both sides of the river, would still be seriously affected by malaria transmitted by mosquitoes breeding in the multiplicity of other pools, puddles, ditches all topped up regularly and kept with fresh water from the frequent showers.

Later, and as part of the epidemiological investigations of malaria and its possible control in Zambia, preliminary parasitological and splenometric surveys were carried out in the Kabwe Rural district, in an area designated as a future demonstration zone for the W.H.O.-assisted Development of Basic Health Services programme. The average levels of parasite infection and the resultant enlargement of the spleen are good indicators of the overall impact of malaria on those sampled. Although malaria was present almost everywhere at this altitude (i.e. below 5,000 ft) its impact varied considerably, being virtually a seasonal diseases in some areas, especially during the long dry season (April to October) and in areas away from permanent water. Under these conditions transmission is mostly by *Anopheles gambiae* populations breeding in the multiplicity of puddles and pools created by the rains but which quickly dry up when they cease.

In this area a residual insecticide spraying programme would be an ideal method for controlling malaria transmission, since it would need implementation only for six months of each year. However, such a scheme would have been costly so it was decided to seek other simpler and cheaper measures. At that time there was no evidence in Zambia of the drug-resistance that had earlier brought the W.H.O. global eradication programme to a grinding halt. So chemoprophylaxis was decided upon – the principle objective being to evaluate the cost benefits of giving chloroquine at fortnightly (at one school) and at monthly intervals at the other. School-children were chosen specifically because they were accessible and easy to follow up and, more importantly, because, although their levels of naturally acquired immunity (built up by constant re-infections) were already high enough to allow them to survive, they would be insufficient to prevent the high levels of infection with its associated pathology, sickness and absenteeism.

The general ages were from 5 – 15 years; they were examined class by class and small finger-prick blood drops were spread on to numbered glass slides, stained and examined under the microscope. Because of the bitterness of the tablets each child was given a boiled 'gobstopper' sweet to follow – a very popular addition – but one that also helped to prevent subsequent vomiting and resultant loss of chemotherapy. Chipepo school-children were treated fortnightly and those at Imansa every month. The results were very encouraging.

Imansa School: The untreated control group rose markedly to 94.9% in March – while those treated monthly fell to 14.6% in March.

Chipepo School: The untreated control group fell slightly, from 57.6% (Nov.) to 50.0% in March – by which time the 47.1% of infected children receiving treatment were completely cured of all malaria infections. Both untreated control groups were finally treated and cured of the infections.

During the earlier prevalence surveys to find suitable schools for the study, the opportunity was taken to answer a question (that had been on my mind for some time); what is the average distance that people walk to the nearest health post when seeking medical aid? To resolve this, three different Rural Health Centres were visited, all in areas away from the main roads, south of the Lukanga Swamp in the Central Province of Zambia.

Sitting beside the Medical Assistant during out-patient clinics each patient was asked the name of his/her village and this was noted. Later these were plotted on a map to which circles of increasing diameters, ½ mile apart and centred on the RHC, were added. This showed that more than 95% of those attending came from villages less than 3 miles away. Later in Zambia I was to learn that a young mother, carrying a very sick child, would be prepared to walk a very great distance (more than 50 miles) through difficult and dangerous country, to seek medical help at the nearest Mission Hospital; though this was probably exceptional.

It is sad to record that the spread of chloroquine-resistant malaria right across Africa and beyond, prevented any wider application of these findings for the protection of these highly susceptible children. At the time of writing, many years later, infant and young child mortalities in sub-Saharan Africa have risen dramatically to over 3,000 per day. For some time now, simple rectangular box-like mosquito nets impregnated with a pyrethroid insecticide, often made in the Far East at minimal cost, have been given out gratis to those living in areas of very high malaria transmission. These initially gave encouraging results but subsequently factors mitigating against complete protection started to become apparent. Although aimed specially at protecting pregnant and nursing mothers and under-5 year old children (many of whom sleep with mum and are protected), when further children came along there would be only room enough for No. 2 – and no room for No. 1. Also, in some cases, adult males commandeered the nets – presumably on the basis that being the main bread-winner, protection from malaria sickness was of paramount importance. This is not entirely true, since adults in such situations will have built up a fair level of immunity to malaria and may suffer only occasional bouts of low fever; by contrast very young children will have little or no such immunity and, if untreated, will quickly develop high malaria fever and many will die.

This completed by first experience in Zambia and was brought to an abrupt halt when I received notice from the W.H.O. that I had been reassigned to work in a general epidemiology unit in Dar es Salaam, Tanzania, led by Dr. Hubert Watson – with whom I had worked earlier on sleeping sickness in the Lambwe Valley, Kenya.

CHAPTER 22

Muhimbili Medical Centre

Dar es Salaam – Pablo the bushbaby

A few days de-briefing/rebriefing in Brazzaville made a pleasant break. The W.H.O. offices there was in a fine new building some few miles up-river at Djoué. We were accommodated in the Russian-run Majestic Hotel, notable both for the excellence of its Primus lager and the size and numbers of its cockroaches, Some of the permanent W.H.O. staff there owned small chalets along-side the river and weekend invitations offered the chance to improve one's aim at boules or sometimes open-air badminton. Brazzaville is or was then completely French – a free and easy atmosphere but also with some general signs of social neglect – many buildings being badly in need of painting and many roads being very poorly lit at nights. The main stores like Monoprix and others were well-stocked, the Air Afrique (Air France) DC8s coming in daily from Paris were fully loaded with essentials – wines, beer and French 'haute cuisine' being high in the list!

The flight across to Dar es Salaam was notable for the 'free spirit' of the pilot who, seeing the clear cloud-free conditions around the mighty Mt.Kilimanjaro, did two fairly close circuits around it for all to see and photograph, before straightening up again on course for Dar. The final approach into Dar airport gave good views of the newly-built Chinese railway linking Tanzania to Zambia and joining the main north-south Zambian rail-line at Kapiri-Mposhi. This was and is an important addition to Zambia's exporting facility – since the routes out to the coast through Mozambique, at that time, were being threatened by the Renamo resistance fighters there.

Dar es Salaam, the 'Haven of Peace' and the old capital of Tanzania is full of character (and characters!) – warm and humid with cooling sea breezes full of the scent of spices making a landfall after crossing some 4,000 miles of Indian Ocean. Its white coral palm-tree lined sands, clear warm blue-green water and its streets full of busy bustling people dressed in coats of many shapes and colours create a wonderful picture. The huge natural harbour is a temporary home to ships from many parts of the world and many magnificent dhows, coming and going from the Arabian Gulf states, continue to trade as they have done for centuries.

The W.H.O. team was housed in the offices near to the Ocean Road hospital which was also the H.Q.s of the Tanzanian National Institute for Medical Research. This has centres in all the main towns and districts in the country where medical research of high quality continues to tackle the many major disease problems. Having been joined temporarily by my wife and three small children we were given a very fine ground-floor flat in a newly-built block at Msasani Bay. This beautifully little coastal inlet was home to local fishermen, who came in from the ocean in their small outrigger fishing canoes (ngalawas) every morning, to unload their catch in front of the thatched huts, built in bush clearings nearby, where they lived. The fish were sold on the spot to those willing to get up early enough – or later sent off to the markets in town.

Soon after their arrival from England, and when visiting the local market in Msasani village with the two children for vegetables and freshly caught fish, a young boy came up to my wife and asked her if she would like to buy a little bushbaby – bright-eyed fluffy bundle wrapped in a small brown paper bag tightly clutched in his two grubby little hands. It had tiny little black paws and two sticky-up little ears. Who could refuse such an adorable offering? Money quickly changed hands and my wife and the deliriously happy children came back to the flat and started to make 'Pablo' (Pl.27) (as he was immediately named) at home.

Being naturally very affectionate Pablo was soon enjoying a lot of love and attention and with quick simian-like intelligence was soon completely 'at home'. Being a nocturnal animal for most of the day he would sleep curled up in my sail-bag on top of the wardrobe. Came the evening he would quickly make a circuit of the flat looking for food and company, both of which were readily available. Once he identified where he wanted to go he would make a prodigious leap, landing neatly on a shoulder or lap, and begin licking one's ear or the backs of one's hand. Whenever a drink was at hand he was quickly in position for his regular sips. Occasionally, if he had 'one too many' such sips he would make his customary prodigious leaps, only to misjudge his landing on shoulder or chair back and vanish down on to the floor – emerging a minute or two later looking perplexed and in need of solace!

Being active at night, when darkness fell he was out on the town but was always back inside the flat, usually curled up in my sail-bag, by dawn. Unfortunately, the flat above us was occupied by a large and overweight Austrian UN Administrator and his wife, sadly not sharing our sense of fun and love of furry animals. These flats all had louvred windows with no protective mosquito netting behind them One night, feeling adventurous, Pablo climbed up and went into their bedroom. The administrator's wife woke up to see a little furry bushbaby sitting on the end of her pillow looking at her expectantly – waiting either for a titbit or a cuddle. He got neither!

Next morning I received a typical Austrian telling off and had to promise to keep Pablo under better control; but like his more famous artist namesake, he had a mind of his own. Fortunately the administrator sensibly accepted my suggestion to press for the installation of proper mosquito netting – mainly as a protection against malaria – but it served to keep our adventurous little friend out of places where he was clearly unwelcome!

My duties were largely undefined and the lack of opportunities for some really useful work were exacerbated by the general lack of transport and fuel shortages. However, the Ministry of Health invited me to join the teaching staff at the newly-built Muhimbili Medical Research Centre in Dar es Salaam. I was given a small office next to the senior pathologist Professor Shaba. He had trained at Edinburgh and was more Scottish than Tanzanian and had a broad sense of humour. Most of my time was teaching tropical parasitology to student nurses, laboratory technicians and junior doctors; the latter in particular were much intrigued by my practice of chalk-throwing when asking questions round the class. These were quickly caught and could be thrown back at me (but only if the answer was correct!).

Soon after my family returned home to England I received a letter from now Professor George Nelson (at Liverpool School of Tropical Medicine) that he and Professor Garnham had recommended me for the M.Sc course at the London School of Hygiene & Tropical Medicine – probably on the strength of my serendipitous B.I.I.T. in the Lambwe Valley, Kenya. This proposal apparently had W.H.O./ H.Qs approval. A week or so later I received a letter from the burser saying that the course was unfortunately already full but that I was the first reserve. This was disappointing; however another letter came from her a week later to say that someone had dropped out and that I was now officially on the course.

With family already back in England I was able quickly to pack up and book a fight to London via Geneva (for routine de-briefing at W.H.O.). I was very sorry to leave beautiful Tanzania with its friendly people and the really lovely environs of Msasani Bay. Most difficult of all was to say farewell to our little furry friend – who had delighted us all for so long with his humorous and affectionate reactions. When I went to fetch him he was deeply asleep, curled up in my canvas sail-bag. I lifted this down gently and carried it out of the flat down to the bay and into the small woodland beyond. Here, being arborial, he would have the best chance of survival. As I opened the bag he climbed up on to my shoulder his warm furry body pressed against my ear. I picked him up – stroked him gently as I took my leave of him ("Goodbye little friend – thanks for your company – time to go home now") then held him up as high as I could reach. He jumped up easily into the tree foliage and was quickly lost to sight. I had to fight back tears as I walked quickly away – back to the now empty flat to finish packing the final few items ready for the journey home.

CHAPTER 23

W.H.O. (H.Qs) in Geneva

De-briefing – MSc course at LSH&TM

Geneva, as always, was a dream come true – a beautiful city with so much to see and do, everything spotlessly clean and highly organised. The W.H.O./H.Qs is a truly magnificent building – almost all glass and marble – seven storeys atop huge marble pillars. The views from the rooftop restaurant and assembly rooms are superb. This stretched out beyond the international airport at Cointrin and, southwards, to the shapely Mont Selève notable amongst other things for its many multi-coloured clusters of hang-gliders. One W.H.O. scientist friend, who lived at the foot of the Selève, flies around the top until it's time for lunch or dinner when he glides down and lands in his own back garden – very convenient!

After de-briefing I was urged to do my best and to make the most of this (I gather) rather unusual chance for further academic studies. I gained the distinct impression that W.H.O. had agreed to support me (with one academic year off on full salary – which was as generous as it was very welcome) but seemed to share some of my own misgivings about academic success; especially as I would be in competition with others far better qualified – several of them with medical degrees and considerable experience in tropical countries in different parts of the world.

During my short time in Geneva I was invited to stay with my chief supervisor – Dr. Pieter de Raadt. Pieter had spent several years working on sleeping sickness at Tororo in Uganda and was, at that time, the W.H.O. Chief Medical Scientist for this disease. He had a beautiful home along the north side of Lake Geneva about 20 miles from the city. We spent a busy evening leisurely analysing the epidemiological implications of the Lambwe Valley work and our associated studies with Tororo. My flight was due out at 07.30 next morning and I was thus somewhat alarmed at being woken with morning tea leaving me very little time to get to Cointrin in time. Unbeknown to me, however, was the fact that Pieter was a motor rally-driver and had recently taken possession of his latest XJ6 model Jaguar. We did the journey with time to spare; I had never before travelled so fast on four wheels – and never since!

Crossing the mountains shortly after take-off the snow-covered Alps in the morning sun were truly a sight to behold; ridges, peaks, glaciers seamed with gaping crevasses, their awesome maws deep in dark blue shade, while the rest were brilliantly lit and sparkling in the morning brilliance. On into Heath Row airport and a train journey back to Devon to join the family for a few days relaxation before moving back up to London.

My older brother and his wife, living in the suburbs, had kindly offered to house and feed me during the year-long course. Apart from the quiet privacy, both of the house and my room and ideal for concentrated study, was the presence of a very active hard-court tennis club at the bottom of the garden – of which my brother was president and serious playing member. The clubhouse was comfortable and, best of all, produced snack meals and had an excellent bar – both essential for an aspiring student! The entry processes successfully completed I moved into the small research laboratory in the London School of Hygiene & Tropical Medicine. On the door was marked Parasitology & Entomology Laboratory; once inside I quickly found the bench space allocated to me and started to mingle with the other fifteen fellow students. These were a mixed bag – from Nigeria, Kenya, Burma, Canada, Australia and a very bright lady doctor from India who, although already medically well qualified was passing the time taking course after course, while her Indian doctor husband was busy working in one of the major London hospitals. She was clearly much practised in the art of passing exams and was thus a likely candidate to come out above us more pedestrian aspirants.

We soon settled into the daily routine of lectures, with much note-taking and practical work-bench sessions, and quite early on we were each asked to nominate a suitable subject for a small research study. This was to be carried out under the aegis of our individual 'guardian angels'; mine was one Dr. David Evans, a tall, highly intelligent and approachable researcher. He was a fine musician, had built his own harpsicord and was also a very talented parasitological biochemist – working particularly on the African trypanosomes of man and animals. When we arrived he had just designed a new liquid solution in which the developing forms of this parasite, usually found only inside the tsetse-fly gut, could be cultured in the laboratory. When this was shown to work well it was immediately christened 'Good Evans' by the staff. Later, when he came up with an even better version, this was of course named 'Evans above'!

For my own experimental work I decided to explore and examine the range and behaviour of cloned trypanosome infections. In nature this is difficult to do since the hosts on which the vector tsetse flies feed are carrying many different populations. To obtain clear accurate scientific facts about behaviour and growth it is essential to study the parasite populations each derived from a single organism. With practice this is fairly straightforward; a number of progressive dilutions are made until, using a very fine drawn-our glass pipette very small drops are squeezed out on to a micro-slide and immediately examined under the microscope. If only a single motile trypanosome is seen, this fact is quickly checked by an independent observer (at one's elbow for the purpose!) and this is then used placed in a liquid warm blood-medium to grow, start dividing and eventually to form a whole new scientifically pure colony – all subsequent numbers of which have come by direct natural division from the original individual.

I explored the School's trypanosome cryobank and since this still contained the deeply frozen and temporarily harmless organisms that I had isolated earlier from the blood of Yemi Daka -who had died so needlessly in the Luangwa Valley Sleeping Sickness epidemic- this was an obvious first choice. In the cryobank there were also 12 different clone populations obtained from Edinburgh. These had all come from a man-tested (i.e. non-human-infective) strain isolated from a *Glossina pallidipes* tsetse fly caught in the South Busoga sleeping sickness area around the shore of Lake Victoria in Uganda. The medical student, understandably thinking it safe to use, was more than a little surprised (as was his supervisor) when he developed a very high fever. He had been infected through small cuts in his hands; he was immediately hospitalised and the quick blood sample, taken at the bedside and immediately examined under the microscope, showed many highly active trypanosomes merrily thrashing about amongst his red blood cells. I obtained all of these 12 separate clones and decided to examine them all in detail – as the main part of my experimental study..

The student had been experimenting with clone No. 10 (isolated earlier from a man-tested (*T.b.brucei*) strain; this clone, when I came to examine it with the B.I.I.T. proved to be fully human-infective. Since this had been grown from a single organism (clone) it showed, almost conclusively, that the trypanosomes the medical student had been working with, was a mixture, some able to infect humans: others not.

This represented another important step-forward in revealing the fundamental variability in human infectivity of trypanosome populations derived from a single organism. For me it confirmed the much earlier eloquent statements, made by Professor Warrington Yorke (of the Liverpool School of Tropical Medicine) in his address to the Royal Society. He said that he believed that this parasite had dual human-infectivity potential – sometimes infecting man: sometimes not., These 'surface coats' antigens are changed at regular 10-day intervals by the trypanosomes, the process being called antigenic variation. By the time the patient has developed antibodies to the specific coat on the invading trypanosome the surface coat has already changed; thus the infectivity element is always one step ahead of the host's immune response until, finally, the continuing multiplication of the parasites in the blood, lymphatics and eventually penetrating into the cerebro-spinal fluid surrounding the brain itself, reaches lethal levels. Without treatment the patient dies and, at the end, the habits become bestial and he/she becomes a drooling, dribbling and drowsy idiot. Not a pleasant prospect but one that makes the early, accurate diagnosis and treatment of this major, epidemic disease an absolute necessity. The vital factors in the make-up and behaviour of this complex and enigmatic parasite, as this is being written (more than 30 years on), are still the subject of elegant and intensive investigations in many major research institutes.

Later in the course we were each given one aspect of a major disease to study and, later still, to present at a special seminar. For this we were joined by a similar group of doctors attending the special M.Sc (Clinical Tropical Medicine) course. The convenor of this was a consultant physician at the Hospital for Tropical Diseases and it was he who led the presentations and the questions which followed each individual contribution. Having been allocated the general overview I was asked to set out the general picture of this disease (toxoplasmosis) in those parts of the world where it occurred. When I had finished projecting the prepared slides and maps – the convener stepped forward saying... "Thank you Dr. Rickman (a courtesy address to all participants!) for that presentation. Now before throwing this open for general questions, I would first like to ask Dr. Rickman if he thinks that this disease would pose any serious problems due to iridocyclitis and choroido-retinitis". "They would for me", I replied (honest as always), " I've never even heard of them!". This produced howls of laughter and much applause – mostly from the medical students in the audience, who probably value such moments of light relief more than most.

The exams when they came were thorough and searching but fair and I was relieved to realise that I knew most if not all of the answers required. The practical sessions were testing – careful dissection of a mosquito's mouthparts, a total dissection of a cockroach (which I finished early and had time to colour all my drawings). The examiners at the viva were Professor Sir Ian MacGregor (a leading authority of malaria and formerly Director of the British Medical Research Centre at Fajara, just outside Banjul in the Gambia) and George Nelson (then Professor of Parasitology at the Liverpool School of Tropical Medicine). Again, the viva questions were searching but fair and presented no serious problems. Thanks entirely to my long and detailed period of initiation in East Africa I found that I had managed to draw ahead of my fellow students, by a whisker, to take the class prize – which was comforting and doubtless reassuring to those at W.H.O./H.Qs in Geneva who had sponsored my candidature.

For obvious reasons I had studied extra hard on those specific aspects and diseases which hadn't formed part of my experience in Africa. One such is the important South American trypanosomiasis (caused by *Trypanosoma cruzi*) with a life history that differs markedly from its African relatives. Transmitted not by biting flies but by Reduviid bugs that live in the cracks and crevices of mud (adobe) walls. These bugs come out at night and draw blood, usually from the faces and hands of the sleepers (hence their 'soubriquet' – "kissing bugs"). Unfortunately this is too often the kiss of death! Scratching the itching bite serves to introduce the trypanosomes into the blood stream; infection is also said to occur when eyes are rubbed with infected fingers. Once in the blood the parasites swim freely for only a short time before entering cells of the heart and intestinal muscles which makes them difficult to find on diagnosis. Pathology includes severe damage to the heart muscle and, worse, the gross swelling of the colon coupled with the paralysis of peristalsis. This manifests itself in a grossly swollen colon – the 'megacolon' – which eventually ceases its normal activity altogether.

Another very unpleasant disease is 'River Blindness' – caused by many small worms that are transmitted by a small strong 'black-fly' (Simulium species – or 'buffalo gnat' because of its humpbacked profile). The aquatic larval forms of this fly need high levels of oxygen and thus are found in fast-flowing rivers and streams – especially where they flow down 'rapids'. Those villagers living near such streams – especially in parts of West Africa are particularly at risk. The adult worms (*Onchocerca volvulus*) produce the disease 'onchocerciasis'; they live for up to fifteen years, tightly coiled up in the skin and causing large nodules. The larvae migrate through the skin and are picked up by the feeding Simulium fly when it probes for blood. When the nodules occur high in the body – around the shoulders or neck, the larvae tend to migrate to the eyes – appearing inside the eye chambers and causing irreparable damage to the optic nerve and permanent blindness. The published pictures of lines of blind villagers, linked together by sticks and being led by a small child, produces the same feeling of helpless sadness as do those of very small, grossly underweight and severely emaciated children dying from lack of food.

CHAPTER 24

Assassination of President Murtulla Mohammed

Lagos – revisit Birnin Kebbi

With the successful completion of the course a request was sent to the W.H.O. Regional Office for Africa, via W.H.O. Geneva, by Professor Lumsden for me to stay on at the School and complete a PhD. This was quickly rejected by Dr. Quenum, the AFRO Director, who informed the School Dean and W.H.O./H.Qs that he had a far more important job for me – one working with the Federal Malaria Unit in Lagos, Nigeria. Yet another quick briefing in Geneva and I soon found myself stepping off the plane into the familiar 'Turkish bath' climate of southern Nigeria. The traffic jams had changed little during my absence and within minutes of leaving the airport we were locked solidly in the midst of a sea of motor vehicles – most of the drivers of which were pumping the horn every minute or so to relieve the boredom. I made two or three shopping trips on foot – each time returning to the same spot. With housing being at a premium I was allocated accommodation in the quiet and pleasant Ikoyi Hotel on the island. Next morning I joined forces with the W.H.O. team at the Federal Malaria Unit under Dr. Ekanem. Our team comprised Dr. Yun team leader and Public Health Adviser from Korea, Dr. Shresta, Malariologist from Nepal, my old friend Gamal Bakri entomologist (who had been with me earlier in Birnin Kebbi) and myself as the Parasitologist.

This brief period spent in Lagos was memorable for reasons totally unrelated to work. One morning when being driven from the Ikoyi Hotel into Lagos by driver Ali we were held up in the usual traffic jam – close to the Government H.Qs building where two separate lines of cars converged before moving on to and across Carter Bridge. As we sat there waiting we heard the sounds of gunfire and, looking across at the joining traffic stream, saw a large black Mercedes saloon surrounded by khaki clad soldiers who were pumping shots into the front of the car. This was the assassination of President Murtallah Mohammed.

"Ali we must leave the car – follow me". We moved to the hedge at the side of the road by the golf course. As we crouched there I saw a small group of armed soldiers coming along the pavement to pass us. Rather foolishly I said to the first "What's happening over there, chum?" Fortunately, he took no notice of me at all but walked pass us, swaying slightly and with seemingly glazed eyes as if drugged. When they were safely past I said "Come Ali – back to the car – don't run. Drive away slowly – look straight ahead and don't look round" All the other cars were as if frozen in time and we were able to move away slowly along a section of the road which was, miraculously, completely clear. "Don't rush" I said, "Nice and steady". Ali, trained during wars years with the army in Burma, was completely composed. But our moving away broke the spell and the others immediately started a mad scramble to get clear away from guns and bullets. It was clear afterwards that the armed group that had passed us were part of the assassination party. A few weeks after this there was a coup trying to oust the army group that had taken over. It was led by a Major Dimka who, when the rest of the army refused to join his small rebel group, fled for his life. He was later caught in a bus crossing into a neighboring country, dressed as a woman and heavily enshrouded. He was tried, found guilty and publicly executed by firing squad on a local beach.

A little later I was called to visit the W.H.O. Representative, in his official office in the Ministry of Health. He said "Whilst you are back here in Nigeria I think it would be very valuable if you were to visit Birnin Kebbi and let us have a detailed report on the malaria situation there; especially of the malaria control scheme, that was put in place when DDT spraying became ineffectual and your team with Dr. Kim was recalled".

I was allocated a small fast kit-car and Ali and I set out early one morning. On approaching Ibadan a line of army trucks was coming towards us on the opposite side. Unfortunately the first truck swerved off the road and hit a concrete culvert. Being large it completely blocked that side of the road. Never ones to miss an advantage, most Nigerian drivers, seeing such a space, tend to pull out of the slowly moving line of traffic, to come racing past and try to break in again further down – by waving a supplicating arm with the cry of "Give chance friend!". Only very seldom are they successful and this makes for some interesting traffic scenarios! Seeing the empty road beside them within seconds the 'chancers' had pulled out of the slowly moving queue and raced down to the bottom – all singing the chorus line "Give chance friend" in order to break back in again. Those so addressed were not at all impressed and kept creeping forward slowly yard by yard, not giving an inch and shutting the door firmly on infiltration! By this time the army lorry, by now back on to the road, was facing a line of traffic as far as the eye could see, with drivers frantically looking for a way back in – but sympathy was there none! I have no idea what the outcome of this debacle was; I can only guess that the soldiers involved would have expressed their feelings in no uncertain terms!

We reached Birnin Kebbi and spent several days there assessing the malaria situation (Pl.28). At that time complete resistance of the malaria parasites to the very efficient drug chloroquine, had not appeared, so the regular dosing of children and expectant mothers with the chloroquine syrup was still working reasonable well. The W.H.O. seemed happy with the report and decided no further immediate action was necessary.

Soon afterwards I received a visit from Dr. Pieter de Raadt, the Chief of the W.H.O. sleeping sickness programmes in Geneva. For convenience he accepted my offer to stay with me in the house on Ikoyi Island to have more time for discussions. Shortly before his arrival a large tug, temporarily out of control, collided with the Carter bridge in Lagos partially interrupting the local electric power supply. The results of this was that, soon after Pieter's arrival and when he was unpacking, the sub-station in Ikoyi became overloaded there was a big bang and all the lights in the area went out. I switched on a hand torch to overcome the immediate problems saying to him... "Don't worry – the lights will be on again in about fifteen minutes or so". No sooner had he finished unpacking, freshened up and sat down to enjoy his first drink, than the lights came on again – bang on cue!

"Tell me, Roy", he said, "In Geneva we're used to the ruthless Swiss efficiency in tracing a fault and fixing it; but how can the Nigerian authorities get power on again so quickly?" "That's easy" I replied, "This happens quite often and I found out that, at the local substation, the huge transformers are on rails and there is always a spare one standing by. When an overload comes the exploded one is quickly pulled back out of harm's way – the points are changed and the new one is rolled into position and switched on!"

CHAPTER 25

John Siwale's Eyes

Join a new multi-disease research unit in Zambia – John Siwale

I must confess to being somewhat relieved when a telex came from W.H.O./H.Qs asking me to return to Geneva for rebriefing. I had been selected to join a completely new tropical diseases research programme (W.H.O./T.D.R) which had been formed to work specifically on the epidemiology and epizootiology of the major tropical diseases in the developing countries and was specially funded by the United Nations Development Programme/World Bank. President Kenneth Kaunda of Zambia got wind of this and immediately made the top two floors of the new seven-storey hospital in Ndola available – for what was to become the Tropical Diseases Research Centre (TDRC). A young administrator John Biles and I were briefed and asked to start up research operations there as quickly as possible. This hospital location was ideal in many ways, being well-appointed with good facilities, lecture theatres and a host of top qualified staff. We were allocated excellent houses and, once all the new equipment began to arrive and laboratory spaces had been chosen and local staff employed, a start was made in designing appropriate field programmes.

Although the Ndola hospital was ideal in some ways, it was very remote from the major areas of disease, necessitating long drives to and from the work areas. Fortunately, thanks to copper, the main roads in Zambia were excellent and well maintained. These were essential for, being land-locked, Zambia relied heavily upon its road transport for both exports and imports – mainly to and from the port of Dar es Salaam (other outlets at that time being hazardous and unreliable). During my earlier experiences in investigating the sleeping sickness outbreak near Luembe, in the Luangwa Valley in 1970, I had made contact with Dr. Herman Buyst, the District Medical Officer at Isoka who had investigated such cases from villages around Kampumbu. Hospital records there had shown that this area was infested with several of the major diseases such as hookworm, schistosomiasis, most of the common intestinal worms, with much malnutrition, poor sanitation and inadequate water supply.

Further, more detailed exploration surveys, in this area at the north end of the Luangwa Valley, confirmed that most of the major diseases were there in abundance. However, although Kampumbu, the focal centre, had a fairly well constructed Rural Health Centre it had no electricity supply and very little by way of equipment or patient comforts; even worse – it was some 500 miles from the Ndola-based TDRC and clearly not commutable. When the small advisory team of experts came out from Geneva a special meeting was convened and both the initial research and staff training programmes were discussed in some detail and research priorities established.

I took the occasion at a programme formulation meeting in Ndola, somewhat diffidently, to throw a stone into calm waters by suggesting that the team concentrate on studying the wide range of tropical diseases present in the Kampumbu region. Also, since it was so far away commuting from Ndola was out of the question. A permanent satellite research unit should be established at Kampumbu with proper housing, laboratory, vehicle maintenance and servicing unit, office with radio link to Ndola and arrangements made for periodic visits back to Ndola for field staff to visit their families; this latter would be linked with a regular weekly supplies and mail run – using the new Peugeot estate car. Since malaria was obviously high on the list of target diseases I added that, during my last visit to Kampumbu, I had caught eighty-three fully-fed Anopheline mosquitoes in a hut where three small children had been sleeping and, also, that the Isoka District Hospital and the Chilonga Mission Hospital (Pl.30), at the top of the Muchinga Escarpment on the western edge of the Luangwa Valley, were both recording a steadily rising number of new clinical sleeping sickness cases.

To my relief this plan was accepted and permission was given to proceed with building a substantial research unit at Kambumbu and also to strengthen the facilities of the existing Rural Health Centre there. For the initial disease prevalence surveys we were kindly allocated one of the local school's classrooms as a laboratory and staff were accommodated in large canvas tents. Before starting to build the more permanent mud-brick houses and stores etc we first had to interview and select the most suitable candidates from the many that, given the poor living conditions and work prospects in the area, understandably wanted the chance to be gainfully employed.

It was towards the end of the hot dry season when the stifling heat of day seemed to crush all living things, driving them to seek shade and lie silently waiting for the cool of evening. Only the cold-blooded heat-stimulated lizards darting about the rocks and the shrill incessant stridulations of the many cicadas, defying all efforts to find them, gave life to the scene. Evenings brought relief, as the earth spun slowly eastwards on its axis and drew a darkening curtain across the sky to reveal a breath-taking display of stars and constellations shining with diamond brilliance down from the immensites of space.

Soon now the rains would come; the clouds were already beginning to stretch up to their full height, inflating themselves with the rising sun-warmed air into magnificent towering castles and anvils of soaring cirrus. These would be intermittently lit up at night by bolts of lightning flashing internally and flickering out around the brooding thunderheads. Periodic releases of the immense build-up of static sent millions of volts in 'trees' of pinkish-blue lightning arcing across the sky and tracing intricate paths among the clouds on their way down to earth – the cracks of thunder shaking the ground and finding echoes in the distant hills and gullies. As they approached, the advancing curtains of rain would gradually blot out the view, announcing the imminence of their arrival with the seductively sweet smell of newly rain-washed earth carried on the strengthening breeze.

As mentioned earlier we were a medical research team, trying to complete the building of a field research station before the rains finally broke and turned the ground into a red slippery quagmire. It was here that we hoped to find some answers to the many health problems that had for far too long afflicted and shortened the lives of the people living here and in many similar situations in the rural tropics. Our earlier surveys had identified the presence of several of the major communicable diseases; together with widespread malnutrition, high levels of anaemia and primitive sanitation these diseases were producing much sickness. This was particularly severe in the young children and in pregnant and nursing women.

Being some 500 miles from our city base commuting was out of the question and it had wisely been decided to build a semi-permanent camp with a small laboratory, stores, vehicle bay, workshop and individual thatched mud huts to live in. It was while we were interviewing local candidates for employment as hut builders, thatchers, grass cutters and general duties labourers that John Siwale first made his appearance on the scene. Even when standing with a group of other hopefuls, waiting to be called for interview, John was particularly noticeable. Dressed only in a pair of blue dungarees with straps over his shoulders and a pair of locally-made 'flip-flops' – cleverly fashioned from old motor tyres – he was clearly a strong, sinewy young man. His lop-sided grin and cheerful demeanour, which found constant expression in his quick repartee and timely wise-cracks, brought chuckles from his workmates and made him stand out from the crowd. But when he came up to the table for interview it became clear that John had one other very noticeable feature – he had opacities in both eyes and was nearly blind. Despite this he was taken on and quickly proved himself to be a strong, reliable and willing worker.

One morning, as I was passing an unfinished hut, where John was sitting upon the roof thatching and surrounded by large bundles of sun-dried grass, he called down his usual "Good morning, Dr. Roy" and added, "would you mind if I asked you a question?"

"Of course not, John", I replied. "Fire away – what's the problem?" With that he slithered down to join me and, with a self-sonscious grin said, "Would you please explain the theorem of Pythagorus to me". Away from the others and despite his smile I could sense that he was serious. Fortunately I had spent the immediate post-war years as a cartographic surveyor with H.M. Ordnance Survey making maps in England; and now, when John spoke to me, I was actually on my way to start making a plan of the camp and had a measuring tape and prismatic compass with me. "Certainly John", I said,"No problem – come with me and we'll work it out together". We moved across to the local school's football pitch and, using the compass and some cut sticks for pegs we marked out a large triangle and then the three squares on each of the three sides. Rough calculation of the areas soon confirmed the theory. We then quickly measured another smaller triangle and repeated the process and got roughly the same answer – confirming the validity of the theorem. When he thanked me and still intrigued by his question, I asked him why he wanted particularly to learn this theorem. He grinned sheepishly and said, "I'm studying 'O' level English and Mathematics by correspondence course and the books I have don't aways explain things in a way that I can understand, and it takes a long time to get explanations back from England."

This I could well imagine; with no electricity, no telephone and probably a very infrequent and unreliable postal service and certainly no reference library, it would be a daunting enough task for a normal person; but to someone half-blind such an attempt at academic study must be like trying to swim the Atlantic! Seeing that I was temporarily lost for words, he chuckled, thanked me again and quickly clambered back up on to the roof to resume thatching.

At that time we had already started preliminary investigations with a view to control a sleeping sickness outbreak in a small isolated village, some 15 miles away. This disease had already infected more than half of the 70 or so inhabitants. Their huts were clustered together in thick bush which was heavily infested with tsetse fies, which carried the disease to them having probably picked up the infection from some of the infected wild animals in the area. Although plentiful in the surrounding bush these animals were shy and diffcult to see in the daytime. To find out which species were responsible we had to dart-anaesthetise them and examine their blood; this was easier at night – driving slowly along the many inter-village footpaths and sweeping the bush with a powerful searchlight mounted on the roof of the Landrover.

Late one evening, soon after leaving camp we noticed a glimmer of light coming from John Siwale's hut. "John's working overtime" said someone with a chuckle. "Let's call in and surprise him" I replied on impulse and drove the vehicle off the road and up to his door. In answer to our hail "Hodi, John" (can we come in?) he shouted back "Karibuni (Come in you're welcome)". We pushed open the door and entered. The hut was very sparsely furnished – with home-made tables, chairs and a straw paliasse bed on the floor. John was sitting at a small wooden box table, the flickering flame from a small spirit lamp (Nescafé tin with a small wick of cotton wool poking through the lid). These lit up the few papers and books that John was indeed working late on – his precious studies! It was a humbling moment – in spite of almost impossible difficulties and at the end of a physically exhausting day's work, this young man was desperately trying to better himself. He clearly needed help.

A few days later I had to drive a new sleeping sickness patient up to the provincial hospital some 120 miles away for treatment. Whilst there I looked in to see the ophthalmologist about John Siwale's eyes. "Yes, we can operate" he said, "The only charges we make are for anaesthetics, drugs and dressings. We don't supply food or drinks – these are usually provided by the relatives, some of whom would have to come with him. We can accommodate a few of them at no cost; in the dry season they mostly sleep on the ward verandah". The cost involved, though modest enough, would clearly be beyond John's very meagre purse – if he had one at all! Back in camp I called John and told him that I had made arrangements for him and two or three of his relatives to spend a week or two in hospital, where the doctors would operate to remove his cataracts so that he could see properly again. Understandaby he was overwhelmed at this unexpected turn of Fortune's wheel in his favour. He shook my hand warmly and was choked with emotion. But the thought of going competely blind, should the operation go wrong, was clearly sapping his confidence. I assured him that the very bad eye would be operated on first and, when that had healed, he could go back to have the other eye treated in the same way. By now I was due to return to England on home leave but, before leaving, I wrote a letter of introduction to the surgeon, for John to take with him. I arranged for transport to take him and his relatives to the hospital and back and gave him enough money in an envelope to cover all expenses.

A month later I returned from leave and, having loaded up the vehicle with all the necessary food, supplies and mail for the field staff, drove the 500 miles to the field station, arriving about midnight. Next morning while being briefed on progress with the research programme, I suddenly remembered John Siwale. "By the way", I said, "How's John? How did his operations go? Is his sight OK now?" They all grinned and shifted uncomfortably, seemingly unwilling to break what I feared might be bad news. "You'd better ask him", they said. One of them went to fetch him and a few minutes later he appeared. No change – still opacities in both eyes. "Why didn't you have the operations John", I asked.

He dropped his head in embarrassment, clearly discomforted by my questions. "I was afraid that I would be completely blind if anything went wrong – then I wouldn't be able to work any more, keep my family and continue my studies". Fair enough, I thought – to be totally blind at this stage would, for him, be an unthinkable catastrophy; but I had to be fair and firm. "OK, John, but if you didn't have the operations perhaps you would be kind enough to give me back the money I left for you" (I would use it to buy large print study books for him instead).

He looked embarrassed and again shuffled his feet. "I can't do that, Dr. Roy – I've spent it" he said, giving me the answer which, by now, I was expecting. "Then if not for the operation John, what did you spend the money on?" He took a little while to answer – as if deliberating whether or not to tell me the truth; then he said "I bought myself a new young wife!"

CHAPTER 26

New Multi-disciplinary Diseases Studies

The Kampumbu field research station in the
Luangwa Valley, Zambia

To assist with diagnosis, treatment and carrying individual patients from and back to the outlying villages the project enlisted two Government Medical Assistants. They were equipped with Honda trail motor cycles with special padded pillion seats and safety straps for carrying patients. Results from the early disease prevalence surveys thankfully confirmed the wisdom of choosing this area as a base from which to work. Snails captured in the local streams were heavily infected and showed two species of schistosomes present, the urinary form (*Schistosoma haematobium*) and the intestinal one also (*S.mansoni*). The collection of urines from children in villages close to these infected streams showed several 'port wine' samples – indicating the amount of blood being passed. This was confirmed later on microscopy by the presence of the large terminally-spined eggs. Several of the faecal samples too showed the laterally-spined '*mansoni*' eggs.

There was also much hookworm in the damp soil around water collecting points (from local faecal contamination) and this, too, was confirmed by microscopy of the stained plastic 'Kato' strips. Microscopy also showed that most of the children were carrying heavy loads of other intestinal worms – the round-worm (*Ascaris lumbricoides*) being the most common.

Malaria was holoendemic, being transmitted all the year round, and sleeping sickness was also present, since the whole area was infested with tsetse flies and there were several species of wild animals in the bush, many of which could be carrying the trypanosomes in their blood. This high prevalence of sleeping sickness in the people and the close proximity of so many wild animals as potential reservoir hosts prompted the joint Sleeping Sickness Research Committee (W.H.O./Geneva and F.A.O./Rome) to set up a major programme to investigate all human and animal aspects of this disease in the Luangwa Valley. One important further consideration for this decision was that of tourism – since the Valley wildlife attracted many tourists all through the year and the several safari wildlife camps there do a thriving business and provide much needed employment locally; they also see that the meat from the game animals, shot under strictly controlled licence, is fairly distributed locally to the sick and needy. The threat of contracting a sleeping sickness infection whilst in the Luangwa Valley, though not a very serious probem, was one that it was felt should be addressed so as not to jeopardise the important economic value of the safari-tourism business.

Understandably initial disease prevalence surveys (Pl.31) by a large internationally-sponsored team of highly experienced and well-equipped doctors, scientists, nurses and laboratory staff (Pl.29), working in the non-electrified rural areas of Africa, stimulated much interest and attention. Once the TDRC base had been brought up to the level needed to process and analyse all the data produced, finalisation of the work-plan for a major epidemiological study was quickly formulated. Now that the working and living facilities were mostly all in place in Kampumbu, the great and the good quickly arrived from Ndola. One large school class-room was made available again as a laboratory (much to the evident delight and distraction of the children!) (Pl.33). Two large patient examination tents were put up – each manned by a doctor and nurse team. The transport section was allocated the task of ferrying villagers from and back to their homes. (Pl. 34 & 35). All medical, logistical and meteorological data were sent back to the TDRC to be put on to the battery of computers, in the hope and expectation of gaining new and valuable scientific findings.

Somewhat surprisingly it was during this period of almost frenzied hyper-activity that many new sleeping sickness began to appear; but particularly unusual was the fact that these new cases were not grouped in any particular locality but widely scattered – ones and twos appearing in several of the discrete outlying villages – an uncommon occurrence. Proven infected blood samples were taken from every case, frozen in the liquid nitrogen cryo-bank and sent back to Ndola for storage and subsequent analysis.

Having signally failed to differentiate the *T.b.brucei* and *T.b.rhodesiense* organisms of nagana and African sleeping sickness, as those understandably dubious of the B.I.I.T.'s accuracy had long hoped to do with enzymes, isoenzyme characterisation now came into its own. All trypanosome strains isolated from the blood of human cases in and around Kampumbu were sent, frozen in liquid nitrogen, to Dr. David Godfrey's enzyme characterisation unit at Langford near Bristol. The samples, some twenty-two in all, had the same enzyme banding pattern as that of a case living in Kasyasya, the first in respect of time. Subsequent investigations established that he was a commercial traveller, born and brought up in Kasyasya, but who was now travelling widely as a commercial agent. He had been taking advantage of a visit home to look up many of his relatives and friends living in villages all within a few miles of Kampumbu and all within the tsetse fly belt.

He had probably contracted the trypanosome infection along the Congo border, where he had been working; whilst visiting friends and relatives locally he was inadvertently infecting many of the tsetse flies that fed upon him and these started a mini-epidemic among the villagers. Fortunately, being on the spot and thus able to diagnose, treat and, most importantly, to have confirmation that all infections were from identical trypanosomes – it was confirmed that these cases were the only ones to have this particular enzyme banding pattern.

It was at this time that the TDRC team received a request from Geneva for the provision of a small publicity booklet describing the various different aspects and activities of this new prestigious project. Each team member was given an appropriate subject on which to set out the rationale and describe what was being done. Understandably perhaps, mine was 'Living under field conditions', since this was relevant to the present and planned research investigations. In the hope that it may also be of some interest to the reader it is given here.

'Living under field conditions'

Longitudinal studies of villagers living in rural areas of tropical Africa usually necessitate the setting up, initially, of tented accommodation, from which such activities as the location and mapping of villages, the completion of socio-demographic questionnaires and the collection, processing and medical diagnostic examination of specimens can be carried out.

Later, if the nature of the scientific findings justify more permanent residence, a more substantial camp could be established which will provide living conditions and working facilities. In planning for 'bush work' in tropical Africa a nice balance must often be struck between the extravagant luxury, redolent of the travelling circus, and the kind of spartan privation beloved by a masochistic minority.

There is no particular merit in 'living rough'; indeed experience soon emphasises the advantages of a comfortable bed as well as strong tables and chairs, all of which can be relied upon not to fold up at unwanted moments. Eating hot food from plastic plates precariously balanced on the knees, in an atmosphere of cosy conviviality, is an image best left in the colourful pages of the camping catalogues. Dining in reasonable comfort with proper utensils makes for a better meal and sensibly avoids the risk of indigestion, burnt knees and gravy-stained clothing.

Good planning at the outset, the willingness of all participants to accept the necessary minimum of camp discipline, facilitates working for extended periods in the field with no insuperable problems. Living 'in bush' emphasises natural circadian rhythms and, since the working day tends to be from dawn to dusk, 'early to bed – early to rise' is the commonsense practice. The African dawn is a daily delight, one all-too-often missed by the town-dweller; and an early start to the working day in the cool of the morning, pays handsome dividends in comfort, output, accuracy and physical well-being.

If those minor ailments are to be avoided that are so often reminiscent of camp life, high standards of personal hygiene must be maintained and sensible precautions taken against obvious dangers. A moderate diet coupled with sound, if simple, sanitation will do much to preserve normal health standards. Toilets must be sited a fair distance away and down-wind and care taken to ensure that there is no danger of contaminating local wells or water sources. Excesses in drinking (especially alcohol) usually result in diuretically disturbed sleep and an 'uphill' day on the morrow.

A good night's sleep in a comfortable bed, beyond the reach of the ravening hordes of mosquitoes, quickly assumes considerable importance. (A long sleepless night, spent in riverine or swampy areas of tropical Africa, devoid of a mosquito-net, will soon convinve any unbeliever of the truth of this statement) while the failure to protect oneself against malaria infection can only be considered a self-inflicted injury, difficult alike to understand or excuse. With the recent emergence of drug-resistant malaria the bed-net becomes an even more valuable friend!

The refuse disposal pit should be deep enough to prevent re-distribution of the contents by wind; also, since the aroma of rotting food scraps is as powerful a deterrent to scientific thought as it is an attractant to flies, such a pit should be sited well away from the camp – and down wind. This will also reduce the risk of razing the camp by fire through the too-liberal use of kerosene when periodically burning off the rubbish. Uncontrolled fire in the bush is an awesome thing and much valuable equipment, even lives, may be lost by a moment's thoughtlessness. A sobering and timely reminder of this was the burning down of two large thatched huts at a field station, with the loss of much valuable equipment, caused by trying to refill a lighted hurricane lamp with kerosene. It should be remembered that strong breezes are often associated with dry-season convection currents and, when the grass is very dry, the carelessly discarded cigarette or match can quickly be fanned into flame – with disastrous results.

Snake or scorpion bites in bush are rare but the risk, though small, is real. The presence (in the camp refrigerator please!) of anti-sera to those types known to occur in the area, will do much to allay the understandable concern of those who, because of their duties, are particularly exposed to them. Under such circumstances the wearing of suitable boots and socks (giving protection well above the ankle) is only commonsense. Those who walk about ill-shod in long grass or (especially) torchless at night, are likely to suffer only stubbed toes or painful thorns embedded in the feet – and not the agonising bite or sting that such thoughtless behaviour invites and deserves!

A small powerful hand-torch, whistle and a pocket compass are useful camp companions; all can be life-savers. It is the easiest thing in the world to get lost in the African bush and few people are skilled or gifted enough to find or keep direction unaided. A mental picture of the general direction back to camp or to strike a road may well avert an otherwise unpleasant incident. Waiting for dusk or, worse, through a long fearful night for dawn, to fix your direction by the sun can be a soberinge experience. Under such circumstances the pocket compass becomes a friend indeed. But remember to remove all metal objects from your pockets and stand some distance away from any vehicle when taking a bearing or you may go still further astray!

For walking after dark the hand torch is invaluable. Ants in particular are no respectors of persons; columns of 'safari' ants resent being trampled underfoot and will retaliate violently – usually after they have travelled all over the body under the clothing. The sudden demented dancing and rapid shedding of clothing quickly identifies those who have stood in or walked through a 'safari' ant column.

Heavy canvas tents tend to suffer badly during extended periods of bush use. They are cumbersome to handle, to erect and to transport. A flysheet provides added protection and reduces deterioration of the canvas through exposure to the elements. The sudden gale-force winds associated with seasonal convectional (cumulo-nimbus) storms play havoc with ill-sited and inadequately secured tents. Both tents and flys should be double-guyed using metal pegs. Where termites abound wooden pegs are quickly eaten away below ground, thereby providing anchorage that is more illusory than real.

Availability of clean, safe water is often a big problem for those setting up camp in bush. 'Boiling and filtering' is the safest course to adopt in almost all circumstances – even where a borehole or deep well is the source of suppy. For lighting and cooking gas cyclinders are easy to handle and reliable – giving instant heat for cooking or light. Locally made charcoal stoves are usually cheap and efficient to use. Their quiet cosy glow on a cold night in bush is an acceptable alternative to a camp fire. But under no circumstances should they be brought 'indoors' – no matter how cold the night. In conditions of reduced ventilation they are swift, potent and silent (asphyxiating) killers. The camp fire, sited well away from the thatched roof huts to avoid the danger from flying sparks is excellent for communal cooking, and one or two large kettles kept quietly steaming in the ashes at the edge of the fire, ensure constant hot water for all purposes.

Opinions differ on the best type of toilet to use in the field. The 'long drop' pit latrine retains its popularity with some but must be well constructed and periodically sterilised with old used engine oil or strong disinfectant to discourage flies. Local constructors tend to provide thatched privacy with narrow and low entrances suitable for 4 ft dwarfs. In sandy soils the sides of the pit tend to fall in, to the detriment both of the latrine and any unfortunate user. The writer infinitely prefers the short walk away from camp armed with a small shovel and toilet roll. The immediate burial of the unwanted is a sure way to keep the flies away! The only problem is that, with time, one has to remember, like a travelling actor, exactly where one has performed before!

Camp refuse is sometimes an inveterate source of flies and the irritating and debilitating intestinal disorders associated with them. The refuse pit should be sited well away from the camp (and down wind) and be dug to a depth of not less than one metre. Burning off the contents is essential; where hyaenas and dogs abound merely burying is usually not enough. Particular care must be taken with old discarded syringes and needles. Children quickly find these and use them for squirting water at each other; the danger of this is obvious and should need no emphasis.

As with snakes the risk of harm by wild animals is usually more imaginary than real. Most animals in the African bush have a sensible and justifiable fear of man and will invariably retire to a safe

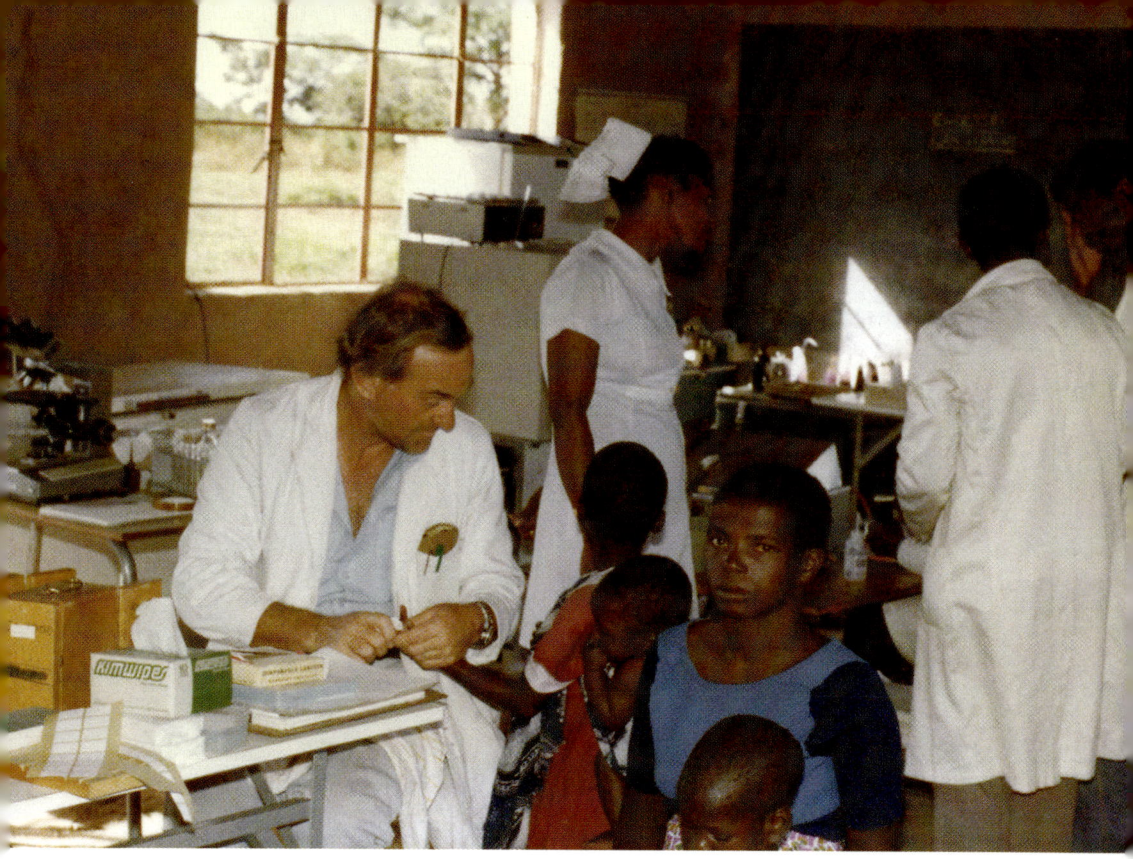

Above: *Plate 33.* Sampling new patients in school-room laboratory, Kampumbu, Zambia
Below right: *Plate 34.* Some bridges need special care (*tenez à droite*)......

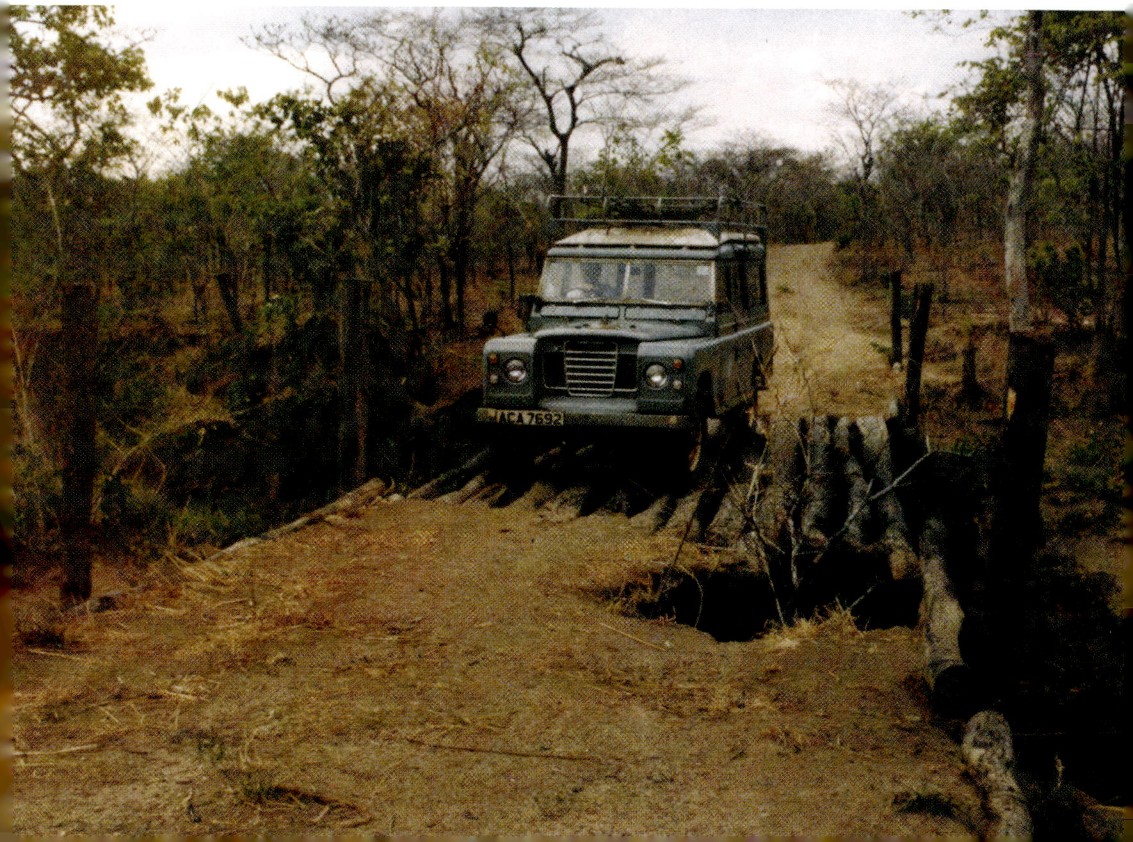

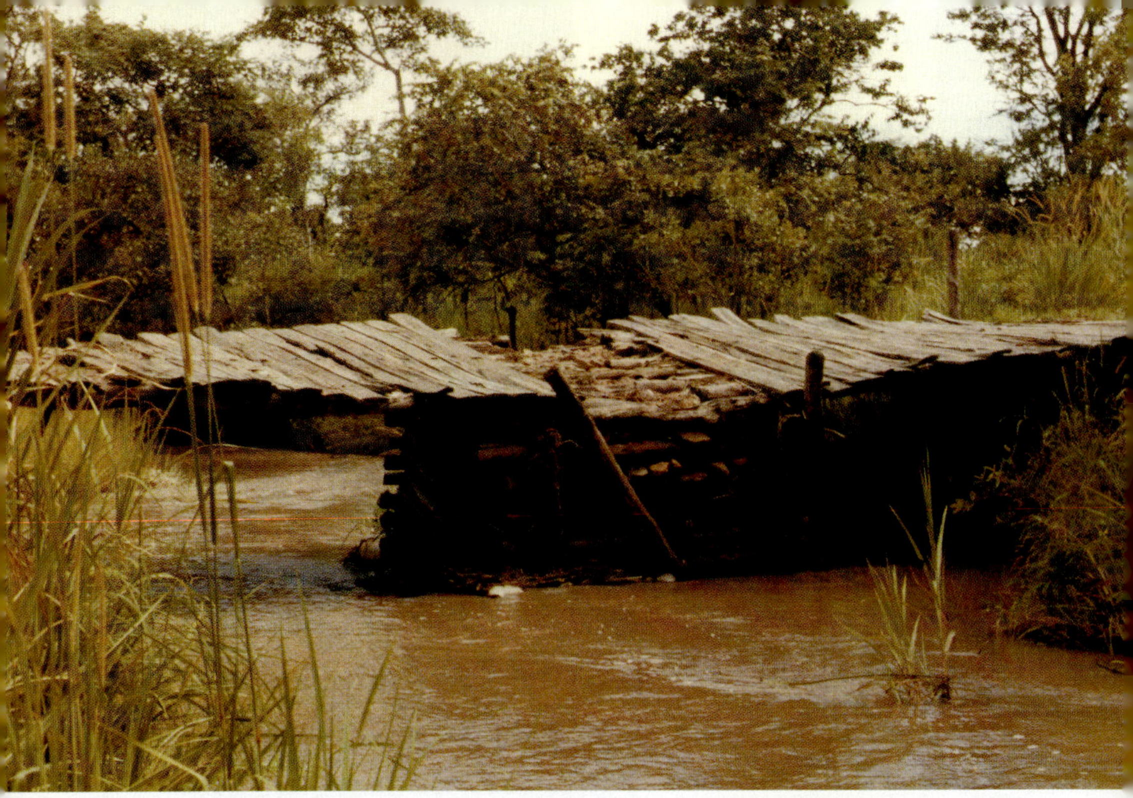

Above: *Plate 35*......others need a good sense of balance, Kampumbu
Below left: *Plate 36.* Young Aquarius, Zambia
Below right: *Plate 37.* The 'Mwanjamwanthu Dancers' waiting to be examined, Mozambique border

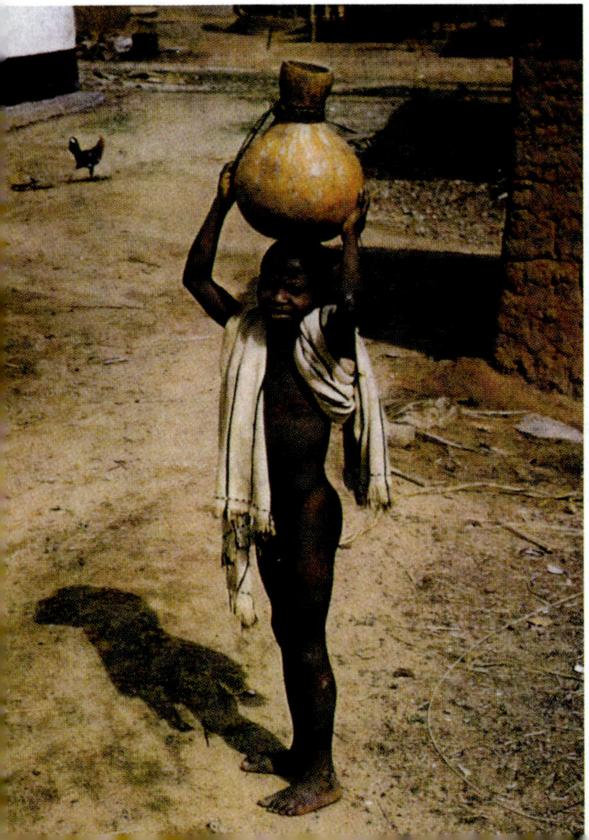

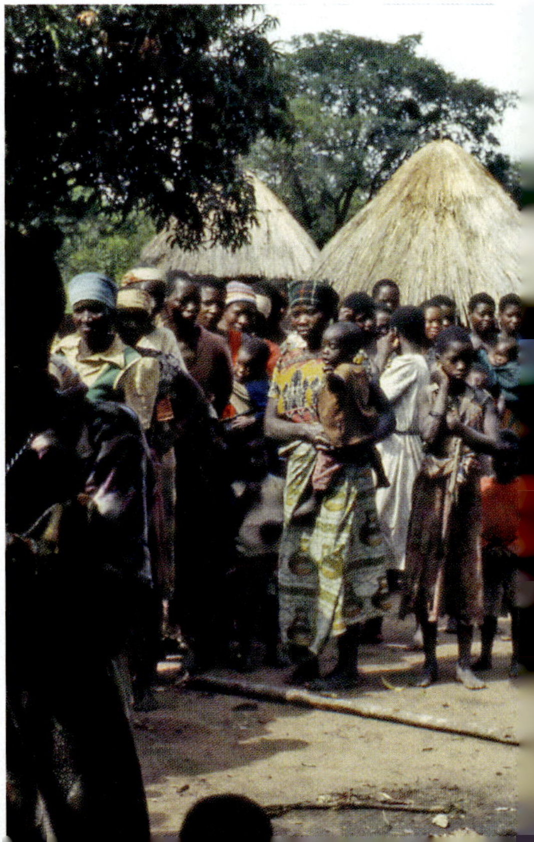

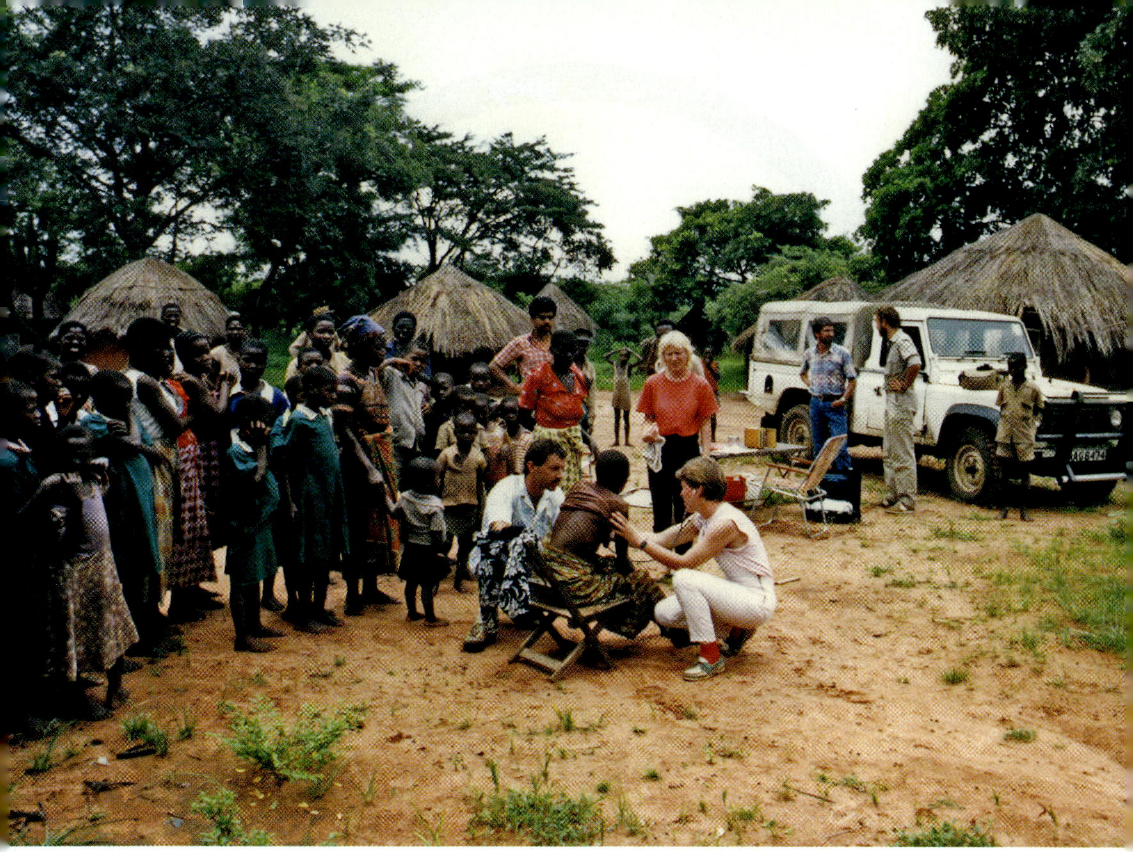

Above: *Plate 38*. Working with the MSF team along the Mozambique border
Below: *Plate 39*. Medical assistant with the 'Spindoctor' centrifuge – for anaemia, Tanzania

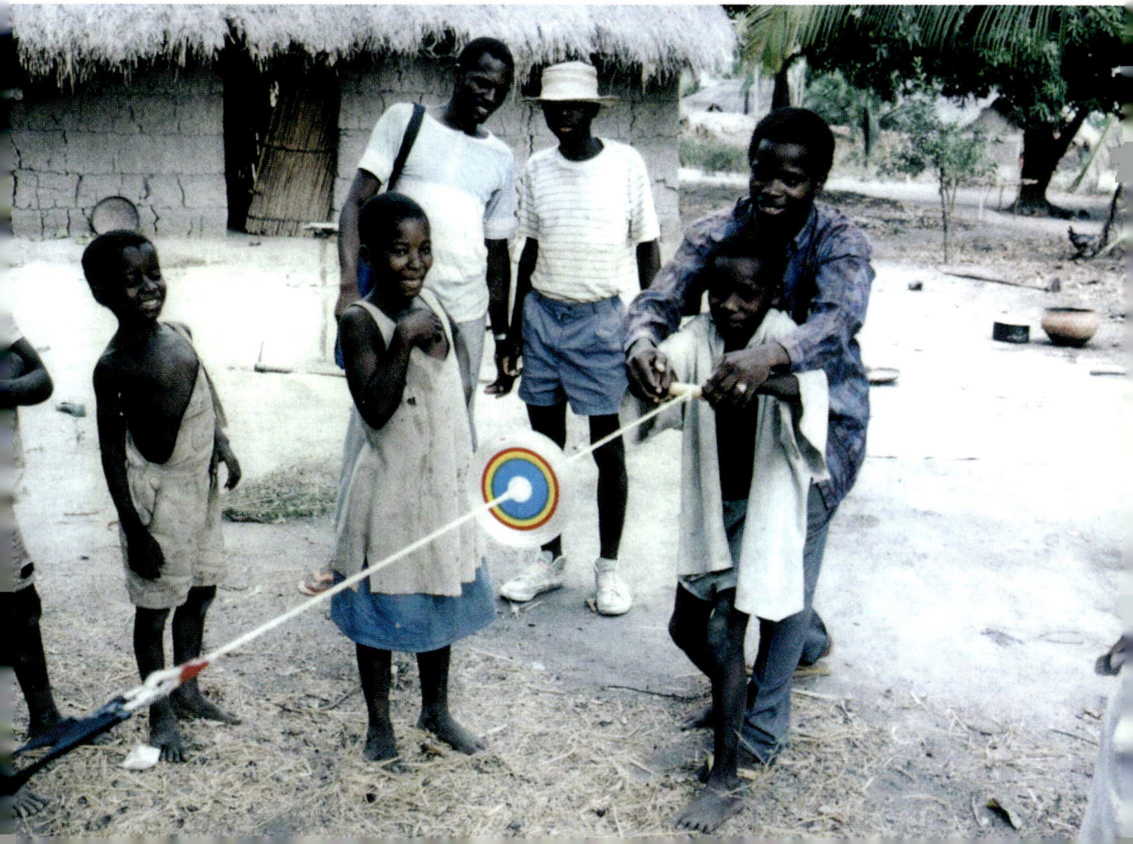

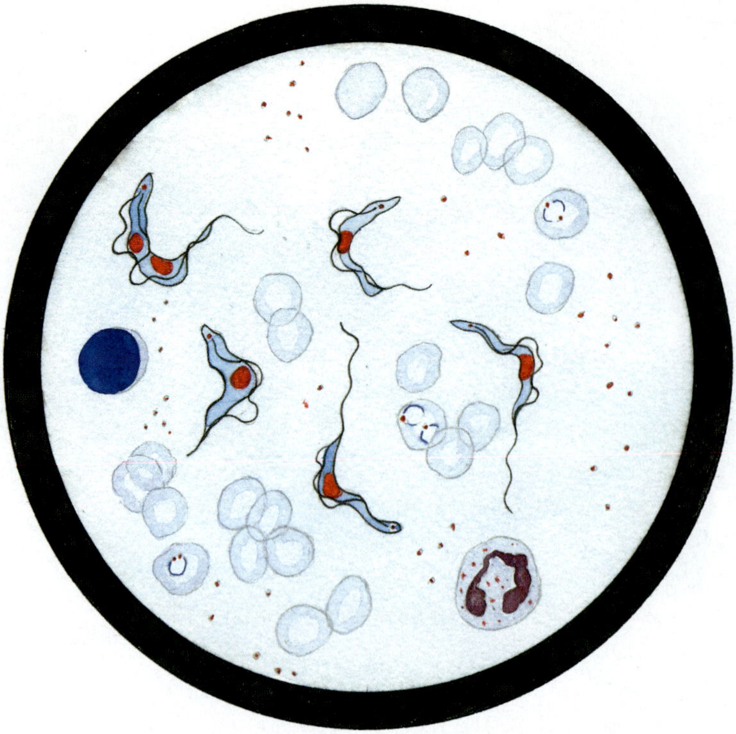

Above: *Plate 40.* Microscopical appearance of (extracellular) African sleeping sickness trypanosomes and early (intracellular) 'ring-form' malaria parasites in a stained thin blood-film.

Below: *Plate 41.* Microscopical appearance of a severe cerebral malaria infection (Plasmodium falciparum) in a stained thin blood-filmer

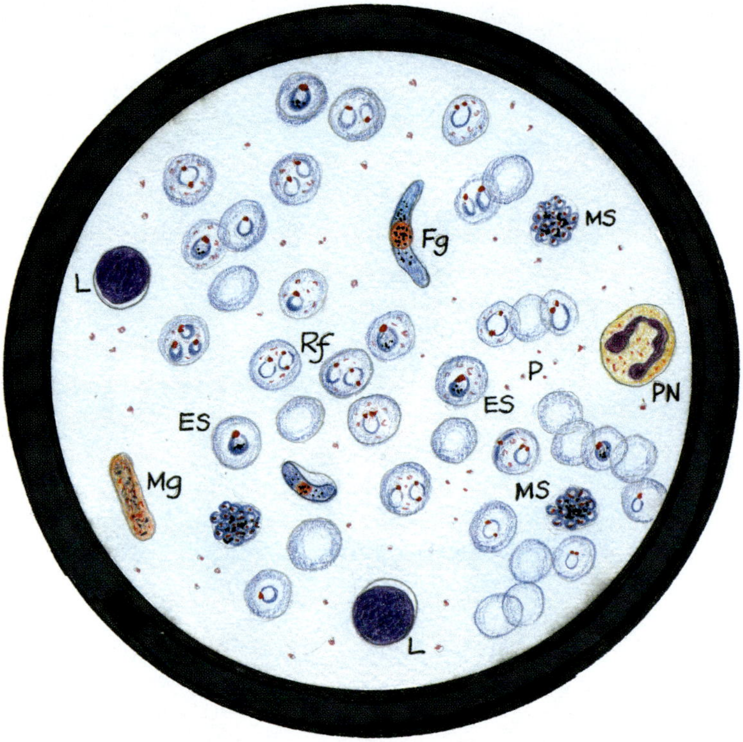

distance at his first incautious (and usually noisy) entry upon the scene. The blood-chilling whoop of the solitary nocturnal hyaena drawn to scavenge the (neglected?) refuse pit, belies its timidity – which is quickly proven by a well-aimed missile or two. However, as with many humans, hyaenas find courage in numbers and very few animals, not even the king of beasts, will stand and face a concerted hyaena attack. Beware sleeping outdoors in hyaena country. Many District Hospitals and Health Centres in tropical Africa can attest the hideous effects of the sudden and unprovoked hyaena bite. Approaching any wild animal on foot or in a vehicle, particularly if it is with young, will often incur the protective attack that such lack of consideration and folly deserves.

Where, through force of circumstance, one has to walk on foot through game country, a pocket full of small stones will often work wonders against the inquisitive larger predators; while a stout staff gives a comforting, if somewhat illusory, feeling of security.

To be free, for however brief a spell, from the clamours of the city, with its incessant demands and dubious palliatives, is satisfaction enough for those fortunate few whose duties take them into the field and who, thereby, come to know the peace and wisdom of the simpler way of life'.

CHAPTER 27

Sleeping Sickness Research in the Luangwa Valley

Working in game camps – saving a driver's hands –
attend ISCTRC, Lagos

We received another visit from Dr. Herman Buyst, the M.O. at Isoka. This time he asked if we would like to accompany him to visit some of the more outlying hamlets some miles from Kasyasya. The track to the small villages of Kayanika, Figolo and Wainga left the road from Kampumbu about half a mile before Kasyasya but was not at all easy to follow. We left the Landrover in the care of driver M and with the intention of making good time we left all portables behind in the vehicle – including food and bottled drinks. Walking quite quickly through the thick woodland we were soon met by a 6 feet-wide band of safari ants right across the road; this we had to jump and woe betide anyone landing in the column! A little further on we were met by a swarm of Africa bees – which all who have experience of these pernicious insects will have considerable respect for them and an innate desire to keep well clear of them. Fortunately there was a small stream a little way ahead which we reached and started to wade through; fortunately the bees didn't follow!

On reaching the hamlets Herman examined all the inhabitants while we took blood samples from those who were sick and dispensed some basic medicines. The journey back was long, hot and very tiring and it was late afternoon when we arrived back at the Landrover – happy in the knowledge that we could now slake our very considerable thirst and have some food. Alas – not so. The Landrover was securely locked and there was no sign whatever of driver M – whisles and shouts failed to bring him in sight. This was not really very surprising when two of the lads ran quickly back to Kasyasya to find M lying in a hut in a drunken stupor. Dashing some cold water in his face and dragging him to his feet managed to get him slowly mobile again. In the meantime – to quench our now raging thirst both Herman and I decided to drink some of the water from a nearby ditch – in the pious hope that we wouldn't suffer more than mild stomach upsets. Surprisingly perhaps neither of us had any after-effects at all – much to our surprise and delight!

Although seemingly still not quite *compos mentis* or fully in command of his faculties, the driver still insisted on driving us the 15 miles back to Kampumbu. It was obvious that he had been drinking heavily and could still hardly walk but, being very large and now becoming quite truculent, it was difficult to reason with him. We covered the first 20 yards in fine style before putting one side of the vehicle into a deep muddy pothole and were stuck fast. Realising that he was now getting near to losing his job, he flung himself into the task of jacking up the rear wheels on to a large flat stone, while the others went into the bush to cut brushwood to put under the wheels for grip.

Luckily I stayed to help the driver and, since it was now nearly dark, helped by shining a torch on the back axle that he was trying to lift. Mosquitoes were already whining around our ears and were a distraction but, luckily I happened to see the whole back end starting to slide off the jack in time to scream at M to pull his hands away. He did so just in time – before the whole banjo casing came crashing down to where his hands had been a moment before. At this Herman decided to walk back with a torch to Kasyasya to summon the 'A' team – i.e. to try to round up enough sober bodies to come and help us. A little later we heard what sounded like a travelling circus – coming towards us – singing, much shouting with whistles and much laughter. The Kasyasya worthies (Pl.32) finally arrived grinning like Dervishes and clearly delighted at some free entertainment to break the normal lack of activity. Herman arranged for them all to hang on to one side of the Landrover – clinging like bunches of grapes from the roof-rack. I selected first gear/low ratio and shouting 'Hold tight!' let up the clutch fairly quickly. The Landrover leaped forward out of the hole as it did so flinging off the human 'make-weight ballast' into the long grass at the side.

We found them easily enough – all lying on their backs and roaring with laughter. They clambered up again and all asked to come with us back to Kampumbu – which would save them a long walk there next morning to attend the local market. Driving back was not without difficulty with four or five sitting on the roof rack and another two on the bonnet. Back at camp they were all fed and 'watered' and put into spare beds for the night.

At the Kampumbu camp most evenings were rounded off by all staff sitting round the large camp fire enjoying a chat with a customary 'night-cap' or two. One night I was woken by a noisy commotion in the next hut. Getting up to see what was amiss I found the three occupants frantically dragging all their beds and bedding outside and coming back with shovelfuls of the still glowing hot embers from the fire and scattering these all over the floor. They had been invaded by a wide column of safari ants ('siafu') which virtually nothing could stop and only fire divert. Any living thing caught in their path and unable to move away would literally be eaten alive – no matter how large. Careful positioning of the embers succeeded in directing them away and 24 hours later there was no sign of them; but every hut that they had passed through had been thoroughly cleaned of creepy crawlies. Nothing living inside that couldn't escape was mere 'grist for the mill' – disappearing into the communal rapacious jaws of the aggressive millions of marching ants.

Once the field aspects of the general epidemiological survey of all people living in Kampumbu and in the surrounding villages had been completed, the specialist sleeping sickness studies were able to continue. Since domestic livestock are invariably unable to survive in tsetse-fly 'belts', those people who choose to build their settlements there are denied the benefits of animal husbandry, i.e. oxen for ploughing, meat, milk and hides and skins. It is a sobering fact that some 4.5 million square miles of African woodland are almost totally devoid of domestic livestock and human habitation due to the presence of the tsetse fly and the trypanosome parasites that it carries and transmits. For example... "animal trypanosomiasis is a major constraint to the socio-economic development of Tanzania. Approximately 60-70% of the country is infested with tsetse flies and over 75% of the cattle population lives in these areas"*

Since we knew that the people in Kasyasya wanted particularly to keep livestock and knowing that goats are perhaps the only domestic animal that can sometimes survive in tsetse country, I decided to put some there – for two good reasons. One was to know more accurately what manner and level of trypanosomes were being transmitted there and, equally important, to see if young goats could manage to build a protective level of immunity sufficient for them to survive. If successful this would at least provide meat and milk for the villagers. The village headman, Friday Sikanyika, accepted to look after them and I promised him that any that surivived after one year he could keep. We bled them for pre-exposure data, and drove them down to the village where they were allowed to wander about freely.

*Dr. C.M. Kihamia et al in Health and Disease in Tanzania, Harper Collins, Academic, London, 1991.

Although a few of them were lost (one was killed by snake bite) some at least survived and managed to give birth to young that had higher than normal levels of protective immunity and survived. Although none had any previous experience of this disease most survived for up to nineteen months there – in the presence of continually high tsetse and trypanosome challenge.

Our work on sleeping sickness was interrupted briefly for a few days, every two years, by our being invited to attend and present working papers at the official meetings on this disease. These meetings were held in the capital cities of different African countries. One of the most memorable of these was that held in Lagos, Nigeria. This was the first time that delegates from Uganda had been able to attend – due to the malignant presence of the Idi Amin regime. The long-established East African Trypanosomiasis Organisation (EATRO), later changed to that of Uganda (UTRO) has had a long history of high quality studies on this disease which has been of historical prominence in Uganda – especially for the work done in the Lake area of Busoga and the offshore islands in past years.

When the time came for the Uganda delegates to make their verbal activities report they were able, for the first time, to give publicity to the extreme brutality of the soldiers and the threatening hazards of their work. They described how the soldiers came to the institute demanding that someone named Onyango be pointed out (Dr. Onyango, a highly cultured Luo African doctor, was then the Director of EATRO). Someone reluctantly pointed to one of the junior clerks who had the same name. He was immediately shot dead. Since any evidence of current work was threatened with serious reprisals from the military and so as not to lose many months of difficult and important work in breeding and experimentally infecting many tsetse flies, all cages were lowered on strings out of the windows whenever the troops appeared. All were saved. The deputy Director, in the absence of Dr. Onyango who had returned to his home in Kenya, decided that the large cryobank, containing many trypanosomes strains from many different human and animal hosts and kept in huge stainless steel tanks filled with liquid nitrogen, must not be lost. They were scientifically very valuable, samples being sent to many different research institutes world-wide for experimental purposes. He loaded them all into a small van and drove them across the border in the middle of the night, away from Tororo and into Kenya – depositing them into the cryobank in the veterinary laboratories at Kabete, near Nairobi. He probably bribed the sentries at the border post, for otherwise he would certainly have been shot.

When the Ugandan delegates had finished describing their work, and the difficulties and dangers under which it had been done, the whole assembly rose as one man and their applause was long and loud at this display of courage and scientific dedication – with not a few tearful eyes at their brave dedication to sleeping sickness research.

CHAPTER 28

'High-noon' at Chambeshi

Completion of major sleeping sickness project in the Luangwa Valley – Kabinga school survey after facing a frightened and well-armed police sergeant.

Once the major epidemiological project had been completed most of the scientific staff returned to Ndola to start the process of analysing the data and publishing the results, together with observations and recommendations for improving the health and welfare of the rural communities living at the periphery. After a short pause a collective decision was made to repeat this multi-disciplined study in a different ecological zone; the area chosen for this was at Kabinga – a village at the south-eastern edge of the large Banguelu Swamp. A large school at Kabinga was chosen as the base from which to work and a large convoy of Landrovers, minibuses and lorries (carrying the large canvas tents) was organised in Ndola.

It was perhaps unfortunate, certainly unexpected, that the war of independence that had been raging sporadically in nearby Zimbabwe for several months, should spread its tentacles far into Zambia. The African guerilla fighters had established major camps, normally in unpopulated areas but all within easy reach of the border. Cross-border raids were common and retaliation by the opposition forces in Rhodesia (as it then was) was usually well targeted and severe, with helicopter gun-ships and commando forces carrying out strategic raids across the border. Shortly before the planned survey of the Kabinga area – a Rhodesian 'nuisance' task force landed at the Chambeshi river crossing in helicopters, sank the pontoon ferry and flew off again. This was where the main road from Mpika to the District capital town of Kasama, crosses the Chambesi river. Thus the sinking of the ferry was a major set-back to the regular traffic in this area. The turn-off from this main road down to Kabinga was only about 100 yards from the ferry and it was guarded by a permanent police post.

After a night's stop over at Mpika the convoy carried on next morning until reaching the Kabinga turn-off. Since I happened to be in the leading mini-bus I said "Wait here a sec ('Ngoja kidogo') – while I go to the police post and check that they know we are coming and that the road is passable". With that I stepped out of the vehicle and started to walk towards the police post. I had covered about 20 yards when a uniformed police sergeant came out and shouted at me "Stay right where you are or I shall shoot". He had a Bren machine-gun slung from his shoulder that was pointing directly at me – his finger was curled round the trigger, he was shaking and was very clearly frightened. That made two of us! He clearly thought that we were another raiding party. I stood quite still and said, as gently as I could, "Please don't be afraid. We are a medical team coming from Ndola to carry out medical surveys in the Kabinga area – and will be staying at the Kabinga school – they are expecting us". My mind was by now in limbo strangely wondering how much I would feel before departing this life in a hail of bullets. "Don't move" he said again – quite unnecessarily. As no-one else came out of the police hut I assumed he was alone. He was still pointing the gun at my middle and his hands were still shaking.

At this point one of the TDRC nurses in my vehicle put down the window and started shouting what sounded like verbal abuse at the sergeant. I turned my head slightly and shouted at her "Be quiet – or else come out here and take my place. The sergeant can then shoot you instead of me!". At this the sergeant smiled slightly – giving me to understand that he no longer considered us to be an invasion force. I said to him, "Sergeant, I can see that you weren't expecting us. Do you have an officer nearby that we can talk to? If so tell me where – then I will walk in front and you can follow me – all the others will stay here in the vehicles until we return".

"OK", he said, "Take that path up towards the ferry – I'll follow you – but no tricks".

We walked up to the ferry and entered a small police hut where an officer sat reading. When I explained who we were and what we had come for he said, "Oh yes. I had a radio message yesterday that you would be coming to Kabinga". Turning to the sergeant he said, "Sorry I forgot to tell you – but please help them all you can". With that we walked back to the vehicles while the sergeant, now all smiles, immediately started to apologise. "It wasn't your fault – you were only doing your job – no harm done" I said, "But let's go and meet the others and join them for some coffee and biscuits". By a strange coincidence it turned out that he was the uncle of a nurse in one of the rear vehicles so, from then on, we were all *persona grata*.

The dirt road down to Kabinga was both narrow and in places had large and seemingly very deep ponds of water on either side, making careful steering essential. Kabinga itself is only some 50 miles from Chitambo – the place where Dr. Livingstone finally died while still searching for the source of the White Nile. He had been hoping that the rivers draining the huge Banguelu Swamp, the Luapula river in particular, would coalesce and drain into the headwaters of the Nile. Alas, this was not so – they join up with the Lualaba river running away westwards and draining into the Congo river out to the Atlantic.

The Kabinga survey was notable mainly for the object lesson of ensuring proper securing of the tents and flysheets. All supporting staff slept in large canvas tents erected on the school's playing field. Unfortunately only stout wooden pegs were used; that this was a sad mistake became apparent on the third night when a strong gale lifted and blew away most of the tents and their flysheets. Investigation later showed that almost all the pegs disappeared below ground – having been eaten away by termites!

CHAPTER 29

The Mwanjawanthu dance to 'Dire Straits'

Survey of Mozambican refugees with a Médicins Sans Frontières team – Wildlife studies – sleeping sickness typanosomes isolated from the brain of a sick kudu at Kasyasya.

The wild game animals of sub-Saharan Africa were always suspected of carrying the sleeping sickness trypanosomes and acting as reservoir hosts from which man became infected. This was proven by the Division of Insect-borne Diseases Division's isolation of a human-infective strain from a bushbuck shot on the Utonga Ridge, Sakwa, western Kenya and another by the EATRO team at Tororo, Uganda, from a local cow.

As part of the on-going sleeping sickness researches in the Luangwa Valley it was clearly fundamentally important to collect as many blood samples of free ranging game animals as possible. It was hoped that this would definitively identify those species that were carrying the human-infective organsims and thus acting as dangerous reservoirs of this perplexing and serious disease – probably in the long-term – athough this was yet to be determined.

For this the cooperation of the safari firms operating in different parts of the Valley was sought. Permission was readily given for the unobtrusive collection of blood samples once the clients had been photographed with their foot on the carcase, presumably gone off to shower, return their pulse rates to normal and top up their alcohol levels! Out of sight and out of mind the blood collectors moved in, took the samples (either from blood vessels in the neck or direct from the heart) and stored these in a small kerosene fridge-freezer kept in their tents outside the main camp stockade.

What they hadn't anticipated was intrusion from an unexpected quarter. The mistake was, in this case, to leave large portions of zebra carcase inside the porch of Salvano's tent. What woke him suddenly from his deep exhausted slumbers was the sudden appearance of two male lions fighting furiously over the carcase. Doubtless horrified and almost out of his wits with fear he ran out of the tent and up to the stockade shouting for help. Fortunately Jan de Coque the 'white hunter' had also been wakened by the commotion and ran out with his rifle and fired shots over the heads of the fighting lions. They both ran off, taking with them the by now blood-stained bed-sheets – which were never recovered (and strangely – which the TDRC administrator expected Salvano to pay for!).

Fortunately, by this time, both Salvano and Gervazious had collected blood samples from a wide range of wild animals so, when they called in on the radio and said quite understandably, that they both felt unsafe, we called them both back to the Ndola Centre – but not before Gervazious had been chased by an irate elephant, to escape which he had to jump into the crocodile-infested Luangwa river. These activities were the culmination of several months of scientific study, working out of two main areas of the Luangwa Valley – Kampumbu and its environs at the top end of the valley and at Kakumbi which was more central – where most of the safari camps had been established and had their game viewing camps and from which they organised the now well-known walking safaris.

For further information on the unique opportunities that such camps at Mfuwe, Cinzombo and Chibembe have to offer, the reader is strongly recommended to read the late Norman Carr's beautiful little book "*Valley of the Elephants*" – the Story of the Luangwa Valley and its Wild Life (Collins, London, 1979). Norman knew the Valley better than anyone… he lived and worked in the region for almost forty years… Here he rescued elephants embedded in the mud and dying from heat exhaustion. Here he lived in partnership with lion, baboon, zebra and buffalo, but here, too, he lost three close companions, all killed by wild animals during the course of their work. This book is dedicated to their memory.

He takes us through the year's climatic changes and the changing patterns of animal behaviour as they adapt to the seasonal changes in the vegetation. Finally, he guides us, accompanying him in the imagination, on a walking safari – to share with him the experience of living and working in one of the most astounding natural sanctuaries in the world. This safari camp ('Kapani') is now run by Norman's friend and colleague Phil Berry – who had earlier been in charge of the elephant and rhino anti-poaching programme in the Luangwa Valley – for which the famous artist David Shepherd had generously donated a 5-seater Bell Jet-Ranger helicopter.

One aspect of our work that was of particular interest to me was wildlife serology – studying and evaluating the natural levels of immunity to the trypanosomes infecting them during their countless bites from tsetse flies. Identification of specific antibodies in their blood (serum) is valuable evidence which can be used to identify the different strains of parasites they were infected with and survived.

Setting up 'Checker-board' B.I.I.T. experiments – i.e. matching dilutions of each trypanosome strain down one side and the range of dilutions of the animal sera on the other. The findings were both interesting and potentially valuable – e.g. sera from hippos destroyed the human-infective *T.b.rhodesiense* trypanosomes as did sera from several bushbucks and warthogs. However, when these were re-tested against a non-local trypanosome strain (from the western province of Zambia) – all survived. This showed that the immunity was local and pointed to these local animal species as suitable subjects for further intensive investigations. Of the 309 free ranging animals sampled in the central part of the Luangwa Valley only 0.9% were found to be carrying sleeping sickness organisms; these were from giraffe, warthog and bushbuck and were identified by the B.I.I.T. as human-infective.

Soon after the closure of the Luangwa Valley project a call came for the TDRC to send a small team to work with a Médicins Sans Frontières (MSF) team, led by Dr. Agnes Croatto, along the Mozambique-Zambia border. The purpose was to examine incoming refugees for sleeping sickness and malaria (especially) prior to their being resettled at Ukwimi, an undeveloped site some 20 miles south-east of the Luangwa National Park in the Luangwa Valley.

It had been reported that up to September 1986 some 17,000 refugees had crossed the border into Zambia – mainly to escape the fierce fighting between the Government-backed 'Frelimo' forces and the rebel 'Renamo' guerillas; by January 1987 this figure had risen to 25,000.

With geographical boundaries being for the most part physically undefined, such movements of these displaced people often pass unnoticed until their congregation in large numbers starts to cause problems which attract the attention of the authorities. Being often of the same tribal grouping and sharing both language and customs, such refugees are readily accepted and may settle easily into existing village communities across the border; but there, unfortunately, they may still be vulnerable to guerilla attacks.

For this reason the UNHCR, MSF and Zambia Red Cross had arranged for them to resettle at Ukwimi – some 100 miles north of the Mozambique border, out of harm's way and where they would become virtually self-supporting.

However, since many of the refugees came originally from districts in Mozambique where both drug-resistant strains of malaria and sleeping sickness had been reported, and were destined to settle in the Luangwa Valley where tsetse flies abound but where no drug-resistant (i.e. Mel. B) sleeping sickness had been identified, physical examinations and the careful microscopy of blood films were felt to be imperative. Another potentially serious consideration was the fact that many of the refugees wanted to keep livestock in their new homes. But Ukwimi is inside the tsetse belt and most domestic animals will quickly succumb to trypanosomiasis infections; in close proximity to a large body of people they would constitute a serious health hazard.

Dr. Lungu, the newly appointed Chief of Mwanjawanthu – a large village settlement half way along the border with Mozambique, was also the Assistant Director of Medical Services in Lusaka and decided to come with us. This village made an ideal base from which to work. One morning a large queue of mostly women and children were waiting to be examined and bled by the medical teams (Pl.37). Whilst I was taking a short break and sitting in the MSF Landcruiser I noticed that it had a cassette player and there was a small pile of discs in the glove drawer. Looking through these I saw one featuring Dire Straits and another Supertramp – both rock bands. Putting the first one in the player, I wound down the windows and opened the car doors widely, turned up the volume and switched on. Within 30 seconds the whole line of women and children were all happily dancing – with broad grins on their faces and waving their thanks – such is the innate African love of music and their wonderful sense of rhythm.

Altogether we examined nearly 5,500 people in 15 different settlement villages and camps (Pl.38) – representing just over 40% of those over 10 years of age. Because of the difficulties in attracting sufficient numbers of refugees to the settlement camps for examination, because most were some distance away busy cultivating next year's crops, examination visits were timed to coincide with the food distribution days – and this produced far better numbers attending.

In September 1984, having reached the W.H.O. retirement age I took a reluctant leave of Zambia and returned to Geneva – as I thought, for de-briefing and retirement. But a surprise awaited me for, athough my retirement from W.H.O. was mandatory, I was asked to link up again with the 'London School' – back where I started. I was asked if I would be willing to return to Zambia to continue overseeing the sleeping sickness researches that were already making promising progress. I was offered (and accepted) appointment as a Senior Research Fellow in the Department of Medical Protozoology (Prof. W. Peters) for a further three years – W.H.O. meeting the cost of my salary.

Once back in Zambia, I moved up to Kampumbu and continued the programme that we had all started earlier – including the sentinal goats. I tried hard to arrange to keep a few young bushbucks there, each fitted with radio collars, to let them roam in the bush around Kasyasya. Since they are territorial they wouldn't be too difficult to locate with direction finding apparatus and they could then be regularly monitored for infections. Sadly this was not possible due to the cost of the radio equipment coming from Zimbabwe and the scientists in the Kruger Park in South Africa.

Instead we started regular night-time sweeps of the surrounding bush using the Landrover searchlight. One evening we picked up 4 kudu antelopes in the light beam; immediately 3 of them ran away into the darkness but one stayed, swaying gently, clearly having balancing problems and standing with its head down. Convinced that this animal was very sick – I shot it quickly and we drove with it back to Kampumbu. On examination the blood showed active (*Trypanozoon*) trypanosomes. Because of its erratic abnormal behaviour I decided to examine a sample from the brain. This was found to be very heavily infected with trypanosomes which were later identified as the human-infective *T.b.rhodesiense* – the first to be isolated from this species. The carcase was cut up and portions taken to the Isoka hospital for patients, the rest shared among the Kasyasya villagers.

It was at this time of closure for the project that we discussed with the Kasyasya and Kampumbu villagers that if they collectively decide to rid the area of the tsetse flies they would probably be able to keep more domestic animals. That most of our 'sentinel' goats had survived and bred normally reassured them that more could be done to improve their standard of living. We advised making the simple screens and tsetse-fly traps, that had recently been designed and tested by the researchers in Zimbabwe, and to persist in seeing that they were consistently deployed in the thickest tsetse-fly bush around the hamlets Some years later I learned that they had done this and had been able both to reduce the tsetse flies to insignificant figures and to introduce some cattle and sheep to accompany the goats – all of which were thriving. This was a tacit compliment to the Zimbabwean researchers, who had made it possible, as well as to the previously stricken villagers who had the courage and determination to achieve such a well-earned success. A ray of hope for the future perhaps?

CHAPTER 30

'Clearly there are many questions – but are there any answers?'

This brief glimpse into the world of tropical diseases research highlights many questions to which, for far too long, there have been few, if any, practicable answers.

The 'Holy Grail' for controlling major diseases is the development and availability of specific protective vaccines. In general, the smaller the disease organism the easier it is to make a vaccine against it. Sadly this has not so far been true of the HIV/AIDS retro-virus – though intensive researches, to find such a vaccine, undoubtedly continue to increase. For the larger pathogens e.g. malaria and sleeping sickness, their capacity for 'antigenic variation' which, after infection, allows them to keep one step ahead of the invaded host's defensive immune responses, presents a formidable barrier to progress.

Vaccine production needs much esoteric and expensive research in well-equipped laboratories, followed by extensive field testing – of both efficacy and safety. Thanks to the beneficence of some wealthier nations and, notably, to the Bill & Melinda Gates Foundation, very considerable sums have been donated to support this research and for making and distributing the impregnated bed-nets that prevent the very young and highly susceptible children dying from malaria.

It is llikely that effective vaccines against HIV/AIDS, cerebral malaria, drug-resistant Tb and sleeping sickness may take some time to perfect and make widely available. But can anything be done in the meantime to ease the burden of disease, reduce the misery of malnutrition, poor sanitation, often inadequate and unsafe water supplies and, vitally important, give early warning of impending epidemics – while waiting for the vaccines?

Yes – in this author's opinion there are several practical, positive measures that would be comparatively easy to implement, immediately effective and affordable.

Firstly, it is of paramount importance for rural health staff to re-establish a permanent physical link with all outlying village communities and all schools by restoring regular (monthly) and effective medical surveillance. Strong multi-geared bicycles would be used for transport and in those areas where there is no Rural Health post within easy reach, the local school(s) would be used as venues for the regular 'Bicyclinics'. These would be very popular, well attended, easily affordable and would do much to ease the present sickness burden of the rural poor. Villagers would receive e.g. diagnoses, accurate treatment/referral, issue of condoms and health education; and authorities would obtain accurate baseline disease data that will be needed to support the later major control initiatives.

A draft work-plan for such a scheme – entitled 'A suggested new approach to delivering regular and effective Primary Healthcare at the Periphery' – is set out below.

Country	% Rural	Country	% Rural	Country	% Rural
		African			
Tanzania	68.4	Zimbabwe	65.4	Somalia	74.4
Angola	66.5	Malawi	76.5	Namibia	69.6
Togo	67.3	Mali	70.6	Ghana	62.6
Burundi	91.3	Uganda	86.2	Sudan	64.9
Chad	76.5	Ethiopia	82.8	Kenya	67.9
Rep Congo	70.0	Niger	79.9	B.Faso	82.1
G.Bissau	76.7	Rwanda	93.9	Zambia	60.5
		Non-African			
Nepal	88.4	Pakistan	63.5	Bang'desh	76.6
Thailand	78.8	Afgh'stan	80.1	Sri Lanka	76.7
India	72.2	Laos	77.1	Vietnam	80.3

Statesman's Yearbook 2004 – % rural populations*.
* Figures abstracted by the author.

Mean % Rural of 21 African countries = 74.0
Mean % Rural of 9 other countries = 77.1

1. Locations

- As the above table shows the majority of developing world populations live in the rural areas. Most of these areas lack electrification – and are unlikely to receive it in the foreseeable future.

- Only comparatively few rural communities live within reasonable walking distance of a rural health post (e.g. 3 miles). Thus, if the rural health services are unable to reach them, for most of the time these outlying villages are medically incommunicado and those living there tend to walk or be carried to seek medical aid only when very sick and often too late to be cured.

2. Facilities

- Almost all outlying villages and clusters of small hamlets that are far from the nearest health centre are within easy walking distance of a school. It is suggested that these village schools could play a vital role in helping to control the major diseases and, through the children, improve community awareness of the health problems and what they can do to minimise them.
- Some rural health services in sub-Saharan Africa are grossly under-funded and have poor diagnostic capability, due to the lack of affordable and better equipment that can function accurately in the absence of generated electricity or vehicle battery access.
- Because of the confirmed prevalence of HIV/AIDS, cerebral malaria, schistosomiasis, hookworm, blood-loss and malnutrition, among many of those living in sub-Saharan Africa, it is considered of paramount importance to ensure that all Rural Health Services have the training, ability and equipment to detect and measure anaemia (Hg(g/dl) and PCV%) at the periphery. The new simple string-powered and the higher-speed (>6,000 rpm) hand-cranked 'Spindoctor' centrifuges (both using the safer plastic capillary tubes for blood collection) are suggeted candidates for consideration. Both have achieved a tested accuracy of +/- 0.5g/dl' compared with routine Sysmex 9000 autoanalyser results, in hospital-based trials.
- Also, without proper reliable transport, rural health service personnel are unable to establish and maintain regular and effective medical surveillance of outlying villages and schools in their catchment areas, especially if they have to cross rivers or flooded areas in the rains. (*See also under Section 3*). 4x4 vehicles are too expensive to buy, to run and difficult to maintain properly. This situation is unlikely to improve with time.
- Due to the lack of quality medical surveillance, treatment that is given at the RHC and later taken at home, is invariably unsupervised and may not be completed. Stopping treatment too soon, i.e. when symptoms start to subside and the patient

feels better, carries the danger of inducing drug resistance and could seriously exacerbate the difficulties of disease control.

3. Prospects for major disease control programmes in developing countries

In recent months much international attention has been focused on funding and supporting specific actions needed to control the burgeoning health problems of developing countries, in particular HIV/AIDS, malaria and drug-resistant Tb. Large sums have been donated by several nations; The Bill & Melinda Gates Foundation has also generously donated substantial funds, to boost the fundamental research needed to produce efficient vaccines against these common killer diseases and supply the insecticide-treated bed-nets.

The successful mapping of the genomes of both 'cerebral' malaria (*Plasmodium falciparum*) and its major African vector mosquito (*Anopheles gambiae*), coupled with encouraging research progress towards a reliable and effective vaccine against this major killer, especially of the Under-5s children, offers good hope for a successful outcome. However present research (in the laboratory and in Africa) suggests that specific vaccines may still take some time to perfect and make widely available to the many millions urgently in need of them. In the meantime there is still much that can and should be done, at comparatively little cost, to ease the present disease burden and provide a sound foundation on which future major control programmes can be laid. These activities would:-

- Re-introduce regular and effective monthly medical surveillance of all outlying villages and schools.
- Provide new, better diagnostic tools, accessories, appropriate medicaments to District Hospitals, Rural Health Centres, Rural Village Clinics and Dispensaries. AMREF Nairobi (Ref: Dr. Jane Carter, FRCP) has kindly accepted to field-test new diagnostic tools and accessories. It is anticipated that this will start later this year.
- Introduce the new 'Child-Safe' mosquito net for Under-5s children, fitted with two no-cost mosquito traps (emitting rising human host odour as attractant) is currently being tested in Tanzania. East net will hold two, possibly even three, small children – to increase efficiency and reduce unit cost.
- Re-establish regular medical surveillance of all outlying

communities and schools, new strong inexpensive multi-geared bicycles (circa $150) should be supplied for all Rural Health Centre Surveillance Teams (each bicycle fitted with the new pedal-powered microhaematocrit centrifuge, wind-up/LED compound microscope with accessories, a dynamo (for night emergencies), puncture-proof tyres and general medical kit). Allowing staff to keep the bicycles, after e.g. two years of satisfactory service, would ensure constant serviceability.

- Provide re-training as required to all Rural Health Staff in the use of the new instruments, in diagnosis and treatment and in accurate data collection/presentation.
- Use regular surveillance visits to reduce the present disease burden with accurate and timely diagnosis to treat the more common conditions, such as sores, wounds, ulcers, and provide dressings and injections as necessary – before, during and after more specific interventions. Vitally important – this would also give early warning of incipient epidemicity.
- Collect accurate epidemiological base-line data to support the later major control programmes.

4. Major disease considerations

4.1. Anaemia

- Many causes (HIV/AIDS, malaria, hookworm schistosomiasis, blood loss and malnutrition).
- Need to diagnose and measure (quickly and accurately), with simple centrifugation of small blood samples collected in new safer plastic capillary tubes. Especially important – check all young children, pregnant and nursing mothers and the aged regularly, both for initial diagnosis and for subsequent monitoring after treatment.

4.2. HIV/AIDS

- Refer all patients with severe anaemia, oral thrush (Candida), cough (Pneumocystis), diarrhoea, weight loss, lymphadenopathies. Treat only under medical direction.

4.3. Tuberculosis

- Persistent cough, weight loss, purulent sputum, haemoptysis. Take sputum into clean sealed containers, send for microscopy and culture.

4.4. Malaria

- Treatment – to reduce risk of further induced drug-resistance it is suggested that ‘home treatment’ is supervised by the local Village Health Assistant – preferably based at the school. This would ensure that all courses treatment are properly completed (many people stop taking the drugs as soon as they begin to feel better).

- If possible involve all school-children in anti-malaria measures by:-
  a) making the plastic bottle mosquito traps (supervised practical school activity).
  b) breeding Gambusia fish (which feed on mosquito larvae) – as a school science activity.
  c) identify and mark all local standing water that has Anopheline and Culicine larvae in it – then either cover with expanded polystyrene beads or seed with fish fry.

4.5. Sleeping sickness

- Regular medical surveillance (with micro-ESRs and microscopy) is essential. The 1999-2001 sleeping sickness epidemic, that spread from Mali to Ethiopia and Mozambique, produced 600,000 new clinical cases and more than 60,000 deaths – due largely to lack of medical surveillance to give the vital early warning (W.H.O. Report). Treatment with Suramin sodium is effective for early haemo-lymphatic infections (i.e. up to 1 month after infection) – later CNS involvement requires more dangerously toxic treatment.

4.6. Hookworm

- Very common and important cause of severe anaemias – infection by worms in faecally – contaminated swampy ground.
- Control by building better water holding facilities with varnished duckboard surrounds, building ventilated improved privies (VIPs) to prevent indiscriminate worm-infected defaecation – if affordable install swing – or seesaw-pumps to lift cleaner sub-surface water.

4.7 Schistosomiasis

- Confirm by microscopy of urine and stalls for blood and large spined eggs.
- Examine and mark all snail-infected ponds and sluggish streams with large 'Danger' signs for children.
- Periodically clear weeds on which snails feed (local labour issued rubber waders and gloves).
- Build and encourage use of VIPs nearby – infection of water by

urination and defaecation nearby (contaminants washed in by rain).

4.8 Leishmaniasis

- Refer suspects for diagnostic miscroscopy of bonemarrow, lymph-node aspirate, nasal secretions or spline and liver samples – for presence of amastigotes.
- Blood culture.
- Control by use of a fine-mesh insect netting.

4.9 Onchocerciasis

- Take and examine small skin snips in saline under low power microscopy for thread-like microfilaria worms. (Take special care not to draw any blood).
- If positives found, search locally for larvae attached to plants or rocks in rapidly flowing streams and rivers.

5.0 A proposed new approach

School extension examination room (and site for regular 'Bicyclinics').

- Although there are many rural communities that are beyond reasonable walking distance from a rural health post, virtually every village or cluster of hamlets has a school. It is recommended that bringing these schools into the rural health service surveillance network would create lasting benefits at minimal cost.
- Where there is no rural health centre nearby the local school can be used by the surveillance team. Temporarily vacating one class room for this purpose causes minimal disturbance and (the author's) experience shows it to be invariably acceptable.
- The school should be equipped with a simple 'Spindoctor' centrifuge* to check children for anaemia (Pl.38) and an inexpensive wind-up/LED microscope with basic equipment for making and examining stained slides. When not needed for patient examination the microscope could be used to improve and extend the school science curriculum. This would serve to introduce all children to basic hygiene and health care matters, at an early stage when they are most impressionable, and lay a firm foundation for better self-help measures against the common diseases. The role of children in local health improvement measures is of paramount importance, since it is they who will best learn them and, later, by guiding their own

children, they will ensure that better health practices continue to be observed and be of lasting benefit to the community.

- Where appropriate all schools should be provided with drinking-water filtration equipment and, if affordable, regular dietary supplementation for those under 10 years.

NOTE: In order to demonstrate the ease with which the string-powered 'Spindoctor' micro-haematocrit centrifuge could be operated successfully by local people in the developing countries, with no previous experience of its use, an initial field trial was carried out.

With the kind permission and cooperation of the Tanzanian National Institute for Medical Research (NIMR) in Dar es Salaam, arrangements were made for a visit to the N1MR field research station at Ifakara. The Medical Assistant at the nearby Idete Rural Health Centre safely collected blood samples in the plastic capillaries (Pl. 24) and centrifuged these successfully using the 'Spindoctor' (cover photo and Pl. 39). Later, during a visit to Makunduchi village on the east coast of Zanzibar, Simai, a shark-fisherman with no previous knowledge of the 'Spindoctor', spun it successfully at the first attempt. (Pl. 25).

A new website will soon be available giving full details of the new affordable diagnostic tools now being developed specifically for Primary Healthcare delivery in the non-electrified rural areas of developing countries. (www.fordcrossbooks.co.uk)

Prepared by: Dr. Roy Rickman, MSc(Dist), PhD, DLSHTM, FIBiol., FIBMS – formerly Senior W.H.O. Scientist (Parasitologist) and Senior Research Fellow (Dept. of Medical Protozoology, London School of Hygiene & Tropical Medicine).

Email: roy.rickman@gmail.com – August 2006.

Epilogue

In retirement I found myself thinking back over my experiences – particularly those in Africa. Prominent among the memories was that of young Yemi Daka (in Chimanganya village – deep in tsetse-infested bush) and George Banda at the Luembe Rural Health Centre. The sleeping sickness outbreak in the Luangwa Valley in 1970 killed over 200 people, one of whom was Yemi Daka. She was newly married, with a new home built by her husband (which she asked me to photograph – which I did and sent her the pictures) and with expectations of raising a young family of her own. But, through fear, largely of the unknown, and despite the almost total lack of medical help available locally, she refused to let us take her the very difficult 46-mile journey across the Luangwa river and up to the Nyimba hospital for treatment. Sadly the well-built Rural Health Centre at Luembe was six miles from her village (Chimanganya). Although staffed by a well-trained, resourceful and dedicated Medical Assistant (George Banda) this facility was of little practical use to Yemi Daka or to the others who died in this small cluster of bush hamlets. It was six miles away; it had no reliable or accurate instruments for diagnosis and it lacked the drug (Suramin sodium/ Antrypol), needed to cure the early sleeping sickness infections and which also protects against re-infection for up to six months. Equally important, even if he had it the Medical Assistant lacked the authority to use it in his rural clinic away from the hospital.

In the period 1999-2001 a sleeping sickness pandemic spread rapidly across Africa – from Mali to Ethiopia, down to Angola, the Central Africa Republic and Mozambique.

It produced over 600,000 new clinical cases with more than 50,000 deaths. The W.H.O. admitted that less than 10% of those living in sleeping sickness areas were under any form of regular medical surveillance due mainly to inadequate budget provisions. Rural health staff are dedicated and capable of delivering Primary Healthcare to their outlying communities and give early warning of a developing epidemic – as here; but to do so on a regular basis they must have better diagnostic tools, affordable reliable transport, the appropriate front-line drugs to treat the common local diseases and the authority to use them. Motorised transport is too expensive to buy, run or maintain so to fulfil the urgent need for regular and effective medical (and veterinary) surveillance it is proposed to issue all rural medical surveillance staff with strong, multi-geared bicycles. These would be fitted with puncture-proof tyres, dynamos (for night emergencies) and panniers to carry equipment and possibly (with care), sick children.

Many outlying rural villages are beyond reasonable walking distance (i.e. 3 miles) or carrying a non-ambulant patient on a stretcher and are thus virtually medically incommunicado. But all outlying villages and hamlet groups have a school to which the children can walk and this could easily be used on one day a month for a 'Bicyclinic'. If necessary some items of equipment or accessories could be safely stored at the school under lock and key, to save having to carry it on every visit. Local villagers will always attend a bush clinic and will also bring their children. If this can be regularised at a static venue, such as at the local school, this would serve to extend the all-important Primary Healthcare delivery with its vital medical surveillance benefits to control the major diseases, give timely warning of incipient epidemics and, particularly important, inculcate in the children an awareness and understanding of the diseases prevalent in the area and how best to avoid them.

Consideration of the mean % rural population figures (i.e. 74% for 21 African countries and 77% for 9 major non-African countries) emphasises the size of the problem and the global need for better transport and tools to provide the vital regular Primary Healthcare delivery. It also served to remind me of the small string-powered centrifuge (the 'Spindoctor') (Pl.25) developed at the W.H.O. Malaria Centre in Lagos and, later, under the watchful eye of Prof. Alan Nunn May, in Ghana. Although this instrument proved valuable for improving malaria diagnosis and for obtaining accurate quantitative anaemia measurements – it was never taken further. Discussing this later with a local precision engineer we decided to start designing and developing a range of new manually and solar-powered diagnostic tools for use in these non-electrified rural areas. Also, because of the burgeoning problem of malaria mortalities in sub-Saharan Africa, especially in the virtually non-immune Under 5-yrs children (over 3000 of whom die every day from malaria) a new small, non-impregnated mosquito net complete with side-protection panels with two no-cost plastic bottle mosquito traps on the top, has also been developed – and currently being field-tested in Tanzania. This seemed a worthy and interesting occupation for one's retirement. To the age-old question "Am I my brother's keeper?" – perhaps the answer is "Not entirely – but to a large extent, I believe, I am". The grossly disproportionate standards of life, life expectancy, food, education, hopes and prospects for a better future – especially for one's children, between those living in the developing countries and the Western World, are now at last being recognised and partially addressed by those capable of effecting the necessary changes. But there is so much more still to be done; so if you, my friend, feel that you might like a part of the action – welcome aboard! As the Americans so succinctly put it, let's go do it!"